YEAR OF THE NURSE

A COVID-19 2020 PANDEMIC MEMOIR

CASSANDRA ALEXANDER

CASKARA PRESS

CONTENTS

INTRODUCTION

What you're about to read is part memoir, part stories from the bedside, and part scathing review of how America pretended healthcare workers were heroes and then made us feel disposable.

Writing this is how I'm choosing to spend my time off after having had a suicidal crisis.

#therapistapproved and no-holds-barred, let's go

– CA

This book is for my husband, who was my covid-MVP, my coworkers past and present, who are amazing and brilliant one and all, and for everyone who ever encouraged me to write this book, both my real-life friends and Twitter-encouragers. I couldn't have made it through this past year without you all, much less made this book happen.

And last but not least, it's for my therapist, Dr. S, who grants me the kindness I cannot grant myself.

PREFACE

On April 25th, 2021 at 10:55 in the morning I messaged my chat group of girlfriends from where I work as a nurse on an ICU floor: "Nothing like feeling strongly suicidal at a job where you're supposed to be keeping people alive," and then tweeted that my "mental health wasn't great" and deleted the Twitter app off of my phone because I didn't want to "overshare."

That I felt like dying.

That I would've rather died than still be at work.

In 2020 there were roughly four million nurses in America. Only 2.7 million U.S. soldiers fought in the Vietnam War.

Those soldiers who came back from Vietnam having witnessed atrocities—and in some cases, participated in them—were changed forever.

You can't send four million people into a wartime-equivalent situation without psychological consequences.

And yet that's what America has done.

We spent a year battling a largely unknown assailant. Running low on gear. Fearing we might bring something deadly home. Getting coughed on by people who pretended that our fights were imaginary, that our struggles—watching people die, day after day, no matter what we did—were literally fake.

Nurses are fucked up.

We are going to continue to be fucked up for quite some time.

And unless there's an acknowledgement and a reckoning, healthcare as we know it in America's going to be hamstrung for the next decade.

I do not know a single nurse who doesn't want another job right now.

Even before covid, burnout levels in nurses were epic. In 2017, 31.5% of those four million nurses changed jobs due to burn out.

A brain drain is happening right now, as I type, as nurses across the nation figure out what safety and well-being looks like for them. Some people will wind up being stay-at-home-parents, some will go into R&D, and others will just retire a few years earlier than they had planned to, because there's nothing like watching people die for a year to make you think maybe you should go and live.

Unless you're me, and yeah, we'll get to that.

And?

A large number of us hate a large number of you. (Although likely not the *you* reading this book.)

If you spent your pandemic fighting masks, voting for Trump, or going on vacation, though? Those of us with the blood you caused on our hands actively wish you ill.

I'm just being honest.

We're going to remember, as we all go into this, our first safe summer.

Because, unlike you, some of us will never get to forget.

This really is a therapy book, and I really was suicidal. But unlike many in my nursing cohort who got through 2020, I am also a professional writer. I don't know what I'm thinking half the time unless I write it down—so I do.

And I kept track of what was happening with me last year. I've gone back and sorted through my personal journals, emails, and tweets to share with you what it was like being a nurse in 2020. This book is going to be a kind of scrapbook, in that I have ancillary material that I'll quote and share here, in addition to my original thoughts upon it.

A lot of it is going to be immediate, and a lot of it is going to be raw.

I'm not here to make apologies about how angry this book will be. I can't, not when that's the reason I'm writing it. Because I need to do something, anything, to quench this ember of hate I have in my heart. Jesus can't touch it, and neither can love.

I need someone—you, if you're reading this—to try and *go there* with me. I want to take you along and show you what it was like. I want to make you feel my fear and desperation.

You might learn some shit along the way—but mostly I just want to not be so alone.

I know a lot of people want to shut the door on the past and move on the future, but to that I say, "How can I?" When this thread of betrayal that this country has woven through me is sewn so deep?

I think this is the only thing I can do that will help to set me free.

And so, now that you're warned, let's begin.

NOTICES

THE FIRST BIG NOTICE:

ALL INDIVIDUAL PATIENT information has been changed so as to be unidentifiable, and no part of this book constitutes actual medical advice.

THE SECOND BIG NOTICE:

AFTER PUTTING in a lot of thought, I've decided to err on the side of readability versus 100% authenticity when it comes to correcting some of my spelling, spacing, and abbreviations from newsletters and Twitter.

While the immediacy that such "accurate" reporting provided felt right, I ultimately decided that I didn't want there to be any artificial barriers, such as grammar mistakes, between my text and the reader.

These changes will be superficial though, and under no circumstances will I be changing the factual content or the feelings behind any of my tweets.

THE THIRD BIG NOTICE

I'VE ADDED the occasional author's note from the present day in the original text with my initials in brackets: [CA].

THE FOURTH BIG NOTICE

DURING COVID I worked in an ICU in the Bay Area. I know I was incredibly lucky that we were never a hotspot in the way that NYC, Los Angeles, or other countries were. That's probably why I had the chance to process some along the way.

My experiences are not meant to be universal to all nurses. Hell, I know some nurses who—mind-bogglingly—voted for Trump. If this is you, please stop reading and go ask for a refund.

What I want this book to be is an acknowledgement of what it felt like to be at the bedside in 2020, accessible to both nurses and laypeople alike.

Nurses—this means that I'm occasionally going to slow down and explain things that you already know, so that laypeople can keep up and learn what it's like to work in a hospital.

Laypeople—this means that I'm occasionally going to cuss and yell like the exasperated ICU nurse that I am. Forgive me in advance. (Or go ahead and ask for that refund.)

· · ·

WITH THAT OUT of the way—if you're still here, book-in-hand, it's either because you want to feel seen or because you want to learn.

I'm hoping I can do both for you, because even though I'm on the sidelines now, I still want to feel like I'm helping.

FEBRUARY 2020

2/26/20—Twitter

Now that Mike Pence is in charge of coronavirus y'all, I am expecting to make sweet, sweet unlimited double time at work any day now. (I'm being sarcastic... but... yeah.)

2/27/20

At my bestie hairdresser's getting teal stripes put into my hair —because if the coronavirus hits no one at the hospital will care what color my hair is as long as I keep coming in.

2/27/20

I pre-apologize, I'm already a very morbid person, even before you add my job on top of it, so if shit gets real, I'm going to get real dark.

Factually dark, as always, but it's going to be pretty gallows humor here.

MARCH 2020

3/1/20

I never feel more futile as a human being than when a patient dies on me.

Two out of three shifts in a row here.

Considering calling in sick for my fourth. When you care for the sickest of the sick it comes with the territory, but still.

[CA: this tweet was prior to my hospital's first covid patient.]

Some quick details about me: I grew up in Texas with my mother, stepfather, and brother, all of whom I love very much, even though things have been strained since 2016. When I was young, we were the kind of Southern Baptists that went to church three times a week—Sunday morning, Sunday night, and Wednesday evening. I loved horses, played a decent violin, and I always knew I wanted to write.

I just never knew how to get paid for writing. This was before the internet, so I'd never met an author before, with the exception of my fifth-grade teacher making us "mail someone famous" and me asking Andre Norton about her cats.

The only map I had for writing as a career choice seemed to funnel into becoming an English teacher, which seemed untenable, as I knew from firsthand experience that kids were assholes.

So, after much thought, my seventeen-year-old and rather sheltered plan was this: to emulate my favorite author at the time.

Michael Crichton.

You likely know him from Jurassic Park—the fabulously popular book and series of movies about dinosaurs genetically engineered from ancient DNA. But his first book (under his own name) was *The Andromeda Strain*—about an infectious disease from space that was being quarantined in a high-tech research center.

As far as I knew—and again, these were pre-internet days—he was a doctor who'd gone on to have an amazing writing career. I assumed he'd become a doctor and then used that money to fund his writing, or that he'd started writing after he retired.

What I didn't realize at the time—or indeed until just now, having looked him up on Wikipedia—was that he'd never actually practiced medicine. He'd written while getting his medical degree, and in doing so had found enough success to go on to become a writer right away. He'd gotten to go ahead and skip to the end.

I didn't, alas.

Life intervened during college, and I wound up in California. But I'd been 3/4ths of the way through a microbiology degree before I abandoned ship, which it turns out equaled about 4/5ths of the pre-reqs I needed to get into nursing school. I applied to my local community college and got in after a stint on the waitlist.

I've thought about good ol' Michael a lot this past year, being that we've all been living in *The Andromeda Strain* to some degree, whether we liked it or not, hell, whether we even *admitted* it or not.

And in hindsight, now that I know he never practiced, and now that I currently wish I didn't, it makes a sort of resonant sense that I accidentally based both my medical and writing careers off of a lie.

IF WE WERE unprepared for covid hitting us at the hospital, then the American populace was vastly less so.

Not only were they operating under the influence of a government that was actively lying to them—a government that some of them had voted for, and in which they desperately wanted to believe —but they were also facing down the barrel of a hundred years-plus of medical "fiction", wherein you watch the "heroes" on your TV solve medical mysteries and heal the sick, over and over, every night.

Your average American has no idea what we do in the ICU— hence them thinking that so many of us were so easily replicable, when ICU beds were running out—and almost every show on TV does nurses and nursing wrong.

I guess cleaning up shit while considering titrations for ten different IV drips after calling respiratory therapy to make a vent change when a patient's arterial blood gas shows their oxygen is low isn't sexy.

I mean, where's the drama in an endless cycle of competent people doing competent jobs?

So in fiction the doctors get all the love. They get to be the moody ones, who have rich inner and outside lives, who get to curse and flail without fear of repercussion.

Whereas on the actual ground, we nurses—in our traditionally feminized profession, all the better to be second-guessed and shit upon—have to hold the line and stem the tide. With our intellect, our physical presences, and with carefully shaved off slivers of our souls.

I NEED you to know that even in the before-times, working in an ICU was all about the denial of the self.

You don't have time to ask for pity—in fact, if you did, you'd likely be mocked. (Unless you've had a really bad day, usually involving the massive transfuser. We've all been there before.)

You're expected to occasionally get blood on your scrubs and piss on your shoes. It is inevitable in your career that someone will try to punch, kick, or scratch you. You will listen to people be racist about your coworkers, and you'll be torn between cussing them out and politely ignoring what they've said, quietly hating them the rest of your shift but taking the assignment, because at least in this small way you can be a human shield for your coworker's sake.

You will listen to the gut-wrench puke-cry of a mother finally realizing that her bright baby has died, and you will get too, too few kudos when someone finally gets to be transferred out the door.

To be an ICU nurse is to understand that being good does not save your life, nor will being bad actually cost you. It is the great equalizer of everyone's experience and pain, and the birthplace of a thousand-thousand nihilists, because to see what we see is to experientially know that God actually doesn't give a shit when you pray.

This job is fucking hard, and most of us do it without complaint, but—let me be clear with you—it was already baseline stressful, pre-covid, and we were all already burnt.

We were just better at dealing with it then. You'd bite your tongue and take your shit home with you. You'd sit in the car a little longer listening to music in your driveway before getting out, you'd plant a few more flowers in your garden on your off days.

But then covid happened.

March 9th, 2020, 10:23 pm
To: my parents
Subject: News Out of Italy is grim

Stay home as much as you can please. I have a gut feeling this is going to get a lot worse before it gets better.

Love y'all –
Me

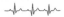

THE NIGHT OF MARCH 9, when I initially warned my parents about covid, was when I saw my first video out of Italy on Twitter.

I do not speak Italian, but I do speak nurse—and all I needed to see was a slow pan of a large ICU where patients were proned (turned over on their stomachs) to know that Shit Was Real.

Your lungs have more surface area at their back. From the front, you've got your heart, liver, and other organs kind-of wedged in there, which you can see if you look at an anatomical diagram of your chest.

But from the back it's pretty much just ribs and lung tissue.

Before I get into oxygenation and lung tissue later though, I want you to know that we never, ever prone people without good cause.

Once we'd gotten the "hang" of covid patients, we would tell patients who weren't intubated (with breathing tubes), who were "only" on high-flow oxygen, to self-prone, so that maybe, just maybe, they might avoid being intubated all together, by using the greater lung-tissue surface area available against their backs to breathe and keep their oxygen levels up.

Proning sedated people is, in and of itself, a dangerous medical procedure.

First off, it's uncomfortable as hell—as any of the awake people we made do it would tell you. No one wants to lie on their stomach all day, much less with a breathing tube in. So if you're intubated (and if you weren't already), we would medically sedate and paralyze you.

The sedation is so that you won't feel pain. The paralytic is so that your muscles relax and you won't fight the ventilator.

The hazard of doing this is that you're totally vulnerable.

Let's start off with skin, as it's possibly the easiest body system to explain: the average person moves eleven times an hour during sleep, if I remember right. It's something like that, because your body knows that you need to move regularly so as not to create the conditions for pressure sores. These happen at spots where your circulation is compromised because the flesh of your body, in places both thick and thin, is pressing against 'bony prominences'—bones on the inside, essentially.

If your cells don't individually get oxygen and nutrients from blood—each of your 30-40 trillion cells, that you, as a human, possess —from your magical, massive circulatory system that touches each and every one of them, they'll die.

Touch your knuckle with a finger-tip right now.

Use some pressure.

See how when you lift your finger up, it's gone white? Because you've momentarily pressed all the blood out of that tiny region?

If you were to keep doing that for some reason, and never allow any blood to return to that spot—those poor starved cells there would perish. Once cells are dead, there's no bringing them back, and as the dead flesh starts to wear away and possibly rot, wounds begin. These are pressure sores.

Compress any part of your body for long enough, and it starts to die.

Now imagine, if you were lying facedown, how many bony parts of your body might be in contact with your mattress.

The tops of your feet? Your hip bones? Your cheek, from where we've turned your head to the side to make room for the breathing tube?

All of these spots would be vulnerable to pressure sores.

So when we flip patients, we nurses know we're getting into heavy care. Because if we don't pad you adequately—if we don't make sure there's no lost saline flush caps in your bed underneath your belly, or a kink in your foley catheter pressing against your thigh

—and if we don't move you every two hours, making you kind-of "swim" in bed by turning your head the other direction, raising your arm, and hinging out a knee, pressure sores are probably coming for you.

In nursing school, I took care of a woman who had had a stroke atop a toilet—she'd been trapped sitting there overnight and hadn't been able to get up. She had a ring on her ass in the shape of the seat, a rainbow of a wound, that I knew would take forever to heal. New cells won't grow if they don't have circulation and, almost by definition, pressure sores are usually in places where circulation is already lacking.

So when you are medically paralyzed, as you are when you're intubated and proned, and when we are the ones in control of breathing for you and feeding you—you're utterly helpless.

Like a newborn child.

And at my hospital, up until covid hit, if you were paralyzed you automatically became a one-to-one. One nurse to one patient, to reflect your inherent fragility.

I just want to get across that making even the mild-mannered-feeling decision of flipping someone on their stomach could have cascading impacts. That happens a lot in medicine.

People are not modular—decisions we make involving one body system invariably affect the others—sometimes for good, sometimes for bad.

Watching that clip from Italian television—I don't even think I had the sound on. It was late at night, I should have been asleep. I wasn't concerned about the isolation gear the nurses were wearing; I mean that made sense, covid was a virus we didn't know much about at the time.

But the fact that their patients were flipped on their bellies, in what is oftentimes a last-ditch, staff-intensive effort to save the sickest of the sick—that made the bottom drop out of my stomach and, for the first time, things felt real.

THE FIRST TEN years of my nursing career were spent in nothing but isolation gear, because my first job after graduation was on a burn unit.

Where I live, you spend the last six weeks of nursing school inside a specialty, shadowing another nurse, and the hope is that you prove yourself there well enough that that hospital wants to hire you.

Of course, everyone wanted to go into emergency medicine. Even me. This was when ER was the world's most popular show. (I mean, if we didn't get into the emergency department, how else were we all going to date and marry George Clooney? Joking-not-joking, in that many people then and now assume that nurses are only nurses to "get" doctors, which is wildly inaccurate.)

But I've always been a little bit of a pessimist. I had good grades, but I was pretty sure the staff at my nursing school wouldn't pick me over some of the more popular kids in class for those competitive slots.

So I looked at my list of options and saw burn on there.

I weighed that in my soul a bit—could I hack that? I didn't know.

What I was sure of was that no one else in my class was going to ask for it.

And if I could do six weeks in a burn center, then I could do *anything.*

I was right.

MY INTRODUCTION TO burn the first night I was there as a student, was helping to take care of a man who'd most likely poured lighter fluid onto an open flame. The fire had jumped back up the fluid, exploded the can, and had horribly, horribly burned him, all over.

He looked like a mummy, wrapped almost head-to-toe in medications and gauze. He had a ventilator and a breathing tube to breathe for him, and six chest tubes, three to either side, to help drain fluid out of his lungs while keeping them inflated. He had a feeding tube so we could feed him, he had a foley catheter to help him pee, and we were taking care of him in the softly lit dark.

He was our only patient. Burn nursing has even "better" ratios than ICU, because the patients there are so easy to kill if they are critical. If a breathing tube comes out of your heat-damaged-and-still-swelling-airway, there's no way we'd be able to get it back in. Your trachea/airway could just swell shut, and while there are feats we could perform to save you, you might die.

So it was mostly me and the nurses I was shadowing (I still love you, B-star! And you too, C!) hanging out with him, and that was when I fell into the ritual of caring.

Every hour on the hour we had to go into his room and get his numbers, see how much urine was draining, and titrate his fluids.

If you have ever given yourself a burn that blistered, you intuitively understand how much fluid can be lost by someone so burned they have no skin to hold it in. A cooking mishap on your finger isn't so bad, your sense of touch blunts awkwardly, perhaps painfully, for a few days—but extrapolate it out. If your blisters encompassed most of your body, that fluid always draining, you would be in very real danger of becoming hypovolemic—basically not having enough fluid volume to function.

Your heart cannot pump what isn't there.

So we knew if someone wasn't peeing enough, their kidneys were compromised, likely because they weren't getting sent enough blood themselves to work properly. Essentially for these patients, low urine output meant they were a quart low, so to speak, and they needed to be topped off appropriately with additional fluids.

I'm telling you this story about my first patient ever because of two covid-relevant things: he was my first liminal patient, and my first experience in significant isolation.

His "friends," who had witnessed the event that burned him, loaded him into a car and dumped him at my hospital's door.

None of them stuck around to identify him, to give us his next of kin... nothing.

So he was essentially trapped in a purgatorial space. Wildly injured, but with no one to advocate for him. We didn't know his wants or desires, he couldn't make them known to us with his breathing tube in, nor did we at the time want to fully wake him up from his sedative medications to talk to him, considering the extent of his injuries. [CA: this was over a decade ago. Lines of thought/care regarding neuro-checks and sedation vacations have advanced considerably.]

And, because of his injuries, because the opportunities for infection were so great, we were caring for him with isolation gear on.

Traditionally, any time someone was more than 30% burned (by surface area) we would wear isolation gear. Your skin is your largest organ—and it's the functional barrier between you and the outside world. It keeps your nice, warm, fluids and deliciously digestible tissue in, and everything that might want to grow in you and on you out.

It's kind-of a gross way of thinking about people or yourself, but getting burned is a cooking activity at its most basic level. Where the skin (and possibly the flesh below) has been burned, that tissue is not coming back, not any more than the chicken in your freezer could squawk to life once thawed. The goals of care as a burn nurse are to assist in debridement of this cooked, dead, likely-to-rot tissue and protect it from getting infected if we cannot remove it yet, while sustaining life to the marginally healthy tissue around the edges of the burn, along with the rest of the patient.

To protect our patients, who were missing vast chunks of a vital organ—we changed into green OR scrubs in our locker rooms, to make absolutely sure we weren't bringing germs from the outside world in, and then before we went into those over-30%-body-surface-area-burned rooms, we isolation-gowned up.

When I started in burn... these were cotton gowns.

I look back at that time and wonder... how. And why. And *oh my God*.

It was not uncommon, at the time, to finish a dressing change and come out with enough blood on the sleeves of your *permeable cotton gown* to look like you'd been in a slaughterhouse. We'd be scraping down dead tissue until we reached the healthy tissue underneath—and healthy tissue bleeds, right? Because it's got adequate circulation! Cells cannot be healthy without blood.

My mind boggles in hindsight. I can't believe we used *COTTON!*

But the goal was to protect the patient against our germs, not so much protect us against theirs.

Over time, these gowns transitioned to plastic affairs, and I don't think I mentioned the other thing about missing skin—people who're significantly burned have to be in heated rooms at all times.

Part of that fluid shift, from the blistering I mentioned—it's from your body sending fluids (lymph and blood) to the affected area, trying to keep those cells alive. (To some degree, this is literally all your body *can* do.) These fluids can cause swelling, which sometimes needs to be surgically addressed, but it can also go straight out of open wounds, where it can cause evaporative cooling. It's like when you get out of the warm ocean on a sunny day—you still might feel a bit cool, as all that water evaporates.

So not only were we in cotton-then-plastic-gowns, with bonnets and masks on, but we were working in extraordinarily bloody situations, in rooms with the thermostat turned up to 80 degrees.

Burn nursing was—and is—endurance nursing.

AND THEN—DO you remember that Ebola scare, when Trump began? When he was maddeningly focused on the improbable chance that some American might get Ebola, and how all of that concern disappeared later on, when we were faced with a legitimate biological threat?

My burn center was in a county hospital located in a major metropolitan area, and we were one of the few hospitals that had actually seen patients with SARS back in 2003.

Because of that, management was tasked with creating a volunteer corps of nurses who would train to wear Ebola-level isolation gear, just in case.

Reader, I volunteered.

I CAN'T ENTIRELY SAY I volunteered for Ebola training out of the goodness of my heart.

Well—perhaps my heart is half-good.

I just don't like the idea of people getting hurt at all. Not if there's something I can do to stop it. I think part of my thought process was this: Why should other nurses risk their lives instead of me? I'm tougher than the average person (I like to think, though it may not be true.)

And if it happens, and I survive, then, *fuck, what a story.*

So I went in for my classes, which were comprised of very carefully pulling on and off bunny suits in a small room while someone else watched.

The job of the observer was to make sure that I didn't contaminate myself or any of my surroundings. She had a clipboard and a pen, and she narrated the prescribed order I should perform my duties as she coached me through.

I did this for an extra 4-5 hours of pay, then the Ebola scare faded, and I never needed to think about it again, really, until last March.

Three San Jose TSA agents test positive for covid-19.
(3/10/20)

3/11/20

My husband and I have an ongoing gag that started when I volunteered for the Red Cross during Hurricane Sandy, about how anytime I come home from something crazy he's just going to hose me off in the yard.

Get the hose ready, baby!

3/11/20

Home and showered after taking care of a suspected case of coronavirus today. Here are my (less glib than prior) honest thoughts, a thread:

FIRST OFF, TESTING SUCKS.

SECOND OFF, TESTING SUCKS.

THIRD OFF, TESTING SUCKS. (etc.)

We've got a suite of suspected patients now, and we're waiting for test results back on all of them. It's Wednesday. We're supposed to get them on Friday. But if not Friday? Monday. ARE YOU KIDDING ME? What the absolute nonsense is that? Here's why it's bad:

In the interim, these patients are HUGE time sucks. Time sucks, resource sucks, staff sucks, etc. Also in the interim, these patients' healths are essentially FROZEN IN TIME LIKE Mr. Freeze's wife. Why? Because we're trying to only do anything with them when we ABSOLUTELY have to.

It's for our health, right? To not tromp in and out of their rooms? But I won't lie, they're not going to get as good of care. And we're also not going to do respiratory procedures to them unless we absolutely G-D have to.

That means someone who only has pneumonia or something else isn't getting as good/frequent care, or as many (if any) respiratory treatments, or getting bronched, and we're not risking extubating them if they might get reintubated, because that puts too many staff at risk.

BUT IF THE TESTS WERE FASTER... we'd be able to do all those things (plus not be wasting huge resources, time, staff, money).

We'd literally be saving lives. But once again the American health care system is robbing Peter to pay Paul, and once again we are paying the price for it.

I suspect I'm going to keep having thoughts, and I'm on for four in a row this weekend, yeehaw, so I'll keep posting them then because I have to yell somewhere. In the meantime, SOCIALLY ISOLATE YOURSELVES PEOPLE. I mean it.

[CA: "bronched" is short for a bronchoscopy—when doctors look inside your lungs for obstructions.]

3/12/20

Just took an Ambien so I can (hopefully) sleep & not be anxious about work tomorrow. Feels like the night before your parents send you off to summer camp, you know?

I've packed snacks and oatmeal in my car just in case.

3/13/20

So the stock market got... 500 billion? And now we're getting just 50 billion to fight this thing????

3/14/20

Oh my God, am I hearing them recommend prayer on this presser? JFC.

LIKE SOME KIND of dumbass going off to war, I also volunteered for covid.

I figured my isolation-gown game was good. I'd had Ebola training, right? (How many people can say that sentence? Not very damn many, I don't think.)

I don't have kids. My parents and in-laws are all sustainably functional elsewhere, so at my house it's just me, my husband, and cats.

And?

Part of me just wanted to see.

I feel like all nurses have rubbernecker souls.

We're constitutionally unable to leave good enough alone, especially in the ICU. Is there something we can be nosy about? Can we tweak this or turn that? Let me look at those lab values again—should I call a specialty?

We are, in a strange way, optimized to provide optimal care.

I HAD this thought more than once on nightshift at the burn center. Working solo in the dark gives you a lot of time to think. In a lot of respects, patient care is like steering a sailing boat. Nursing gives you the opportunity to be in charge of your own ship, and sometimes, given how rowdy nurses can be, your very own pirate crew (she says with love). A heart rate drifts up, you give medication to push it back down. A blood pressure goes low, and you titrate an IV drip up.

You fuss and you finesse, and if all goes well and the patient agrees to live (metaphorically and sometimes literally), you can steer them through the Scylla of sepsis and the Charybdis of cardiac arrest and maybe, just maybe, everything turns out all right.

They make it out of the critical zone, they get downgraded to another floor, they possibly take a detour to rehab, and then they go home.

That's the goal, at least.

It is always—almost always—the goal.

And at all points along the way as a nurse, you feel like you are doing something to make that happen.

Because no one comes up to the ICU to coast.

You're there because some bodily system is horribly out of whack, and only continuous, present, thoughtful care can get you through.

People make a big deal about doctors, and yes, they have very important jobs, and no, despite my original scholastic intentions, I am very glad not to be one.

But they oftentimes just play a navigator's role in a patient's care. They learn where the patient *is* and demarcate where they want them to *be*.

It is the bedside nursing that actually gets you there. Our hands are on the pumps and ventilators (alongside the respiratory therapist's). We work within the parameters we've been given and the years of cumulative experience on our floor—not just in our own minds, as we frequently ask one another questions—to move you from point A to point B.

And we do nothing without purpose, no matter how humble it may seem.

We brush your teeth for you, because you cannot—and because doing it every four hours on an intubated patient reduces the germ-load and subsequent chances of getting ventilator-associated pneumonia. We wipe your ass for you, because you cannot—because sitting in wetness of any sort is likely to give you sores.

Everything we do is in an attempt to heal you.

Is it a calling? Or just a refuge for anal-retentive perfectionists who enjoy bossing people around?

Possibly both. I won't lie.

But no matter how we get there, our intentions are always good.

And none of us ever want to see people suffer or die. A patient may come *in* like that, but that's not how we want them to *be*.

That's not what we signed up for.

3/14/20—tweets made while walking from my car into work

Some staff refused assignments this morning and walked out. We have an active case and many more tests pending. (These are not ICU RNs, mind you—the gossip just percolated to my floor.)

That is the problem with calling us heroes. I honestly can't blame those RNs. Shit's scary.

I'm not going anywhere though. I came in early on Weds to volunteer to take any active cases. No kids, no nearby elderly in my life.

But I'm also not a hero.

I'm a hyper-intelligent malcontent who likes to be in the middle of shit. Always have, always will.

I have a bitty death wish too (as my role-playing-game friends can attest.)

So I'm in this till it's through.

Also, if I survive this, I am getting my hair done in mermaid rainbow colors and nobody better say shit to me for years.

Excerpt from a retrospective journal, written 3/14/2021, but written about 3/14/2020.

...during that working stretch I had two possible covid patients. This was before rapid testing, when we'd run through gear for days before we'd find out if someone actually had it or not.

One of my patients was awake and watching the television and getting frustrated that they were living out *The Andromeda Strain*.

The other was intubated and not doing so hot.

They were both in negative-pressure isolation rooms with a little antechamber full of isolation gear between them. We didn't know then that a gear shortage was right around the corner. It'd never even occurred to us we might run out. This was back when we still had shields for our CAPRs—positive pressure breathing helmets that wrapped around your face and cleaned your air for you—back when we still thought said-shields should be disposable, rather than reused all day, every day, for multiple shifts, just wiped down in between with bleach wipes.

(You will never convince me that the scent of bleach is not safety. From here on out, for the rest of my life, I will have a visceral scent association that bleach is good.)

The awake person was pretty pissed, actually. They were a long-term smoker and their nicotine patch wasn't cutting it. They were on oxygen at home and had COPD. They didn't understand why we were acting like they were an alien. They were cranky and hungry and we weren't letting them eat because we were worried we might have to intubate them. I think they were mad at us because we were treating them weird and I'm sure it was scary.

I wish I could say that I was totally fearless in there, but I was not.

Just because I always kinda-sorta-itty-bitty wanna die doesn't mean that I want to die right-now-this-very-moment.

So while I put on a good game because I'm nothing if not adept at hiding my emotions (when I feel like it), a part of me was still, "Why the fuckkkkkkk did we do this to ourselves, Casssssiiieeeeee. You have so much to live fooooooorrrrr and so many books to writtteeeee."

And they're hacking with their smoker's cough, and all I can see is what I think of as germs billowing out of their mouth and plastering themselves against the outside of my shield's plastic screen, covering me up in a fine film of death-mist.

Eventually our doctors decide they're not going to intubate them, not today at least, so they can finally have some dinner, and I brought it in with me.

When patients are on isolation you don't take anything back out of their rooms. Even their food comes in on disposable trays. I'm trying to air-lock-seal the door behind me so everything they're coughing doesn't get into my antechamber, while holding a flimsy cardboard tray, while my hands are shaking probably—and I dump their whole food tray on the floor.

We both watch it fall.

The food they've been waiting for, for two days, just gone, splat.

And of course it makes a mess everywhere, which I now have to clean up, and they start yelling at me and I start apologizing because I do feel like an asshole, but there's nothing I can do. I get it clean, I hop out of their room, and I order them more, and then I go hide in my other patient's room, who, while notably sicker, is at least not yelling at me, because he's intubated and all.

I'm in there, doing something-something patient care, I don't really remember.

What I do remember clearly is my coworker, coming over to rap on the glass door with her fist. She gets my attention and then she holds her hands and crosses them into a plus-sign.

He's positive.

For reals.

I'm in there with him.

And the fear of the still-possibly-imaginary-death-mist of my other patient evaporates as I realize I'm actually in the presence of it now, one hundred percent legitimately.

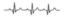

IT'S EASIER to nurse when there's no one watching, that's for sure. No one listening to you when you talk to yourself behind your mask, psyching yourself up to do what needs doing.

I think that's one of the reasons I like ICU, as opposed to other forms of nursing with more "lively" patients. It's a lot easier to be crazy, because your patients aren't usually awake enough to care, as long as their outcomes are good (as can be expected, given the scenario).

So as long as no one's crashing, you can stand in the corner of a room for quite some time if you need to, with the lights off even, in the dark, sorting your shit out before it's go-time. If you only knew how many nights I cried through shifts due to personal stuff and my own brain-hating me, with only the bodies of the patients I gently steered away from mortal reefs as witness. And a lot of the time, when you're nursing, you're too busy to worry about your own shit, which makes it a really good occupation for me, seeing as "getting too up in my own head" is a perennial danger. (I am admitting to this here because I know enough other nurses have also nursed like this as well. Surprise! The people who care for you at your darkest hours are still human and not robots.)

Now that we knew he was positive, it wasn't like anyone else wanted to come into the room with me, besides.

Nor would I have let them. You should've seen the contortions we went through in those days to make absolutely sure there was no reason for any other person or service to go into the positive rooms. We left nothing for the break nurses to do if at all possible. Just think of how badly we want to keep you safe—we wanted to keep our coworkers a thousand-times safer. And you should've also seen how the doctors were back then, standing outside the glass, peering in, shouting instructions at you, rather than coming into the rooms themselves.... I couldn't entirely blame them, but more than one of them had the gall to call us brave because we were physically in the room with the patients, like we had a choice—like they apparently did.

I did my job and kept swimming that day, and the next. I think our tests were running 4-5 days then? And I hadn't taken back my offer to volunteer for covid patients because I'm stupidly stubborn like that (so I lived on the covid wing for months).

I got my pair of patients back after a day off, and it turned out that the smoker didn't have covid. I got to be the one to tell them, and they were ecstatic about it. We talked about things—like, that particular week in March was when shit really started hitting the fan, and they'd been watching the news that whole time, so our fears for them seemed really legitimate. It'd all sunk in, and they really were scared. They couldn't wait to go home and go back to their life.

And me, I was thinking, "Wow. They're one of the few people in the US right now who actually knows that they don't have covid— and the second they leave here, they can't be sure of that anymore, really."

I did try to impress that on them, that just because they'd had a negative test, it was just a snapshot of a moment, and it didn't mean they'd be safe for an extended period of time.

They promised me they understood.

Meanwhile my other intubated patient... got better?

Like, way better.

Eventually we extubated him successfully.

This was before we knew how shitty the chances of that really were.

To us it seemed like a given. I mean, he was in his 30s, quite healthy in all other respects.

It was kind-of cheating to get a win so early in the game. It let me think that wins were possible, and it really set my expectations out of whack.

When we extubated him he'd been under for seven days, so it was like talking to a time traveler. He had no idea what'd happened to him, whereas I got to talk to him about the world's nev problems.

Turns out he was a competitive athlete. He credited that for making his lungs strong. It seemed a good enough reason as any—I was just glad he was alive, although I'd learn soon after that how much I couldn't take anything covid-related for granted.

We were getting more cases; things were ramping up and people were starting to lock down and... well... you all know the rest.

3/14/20

Heard management talking to my favorite doctor on my way out: "It's not if we run out of supplies, it's when."

While I knew this was going to suck intellectually, this is kind the first time I've felt it emotionally.

I wonder if this is how soldiers felt in WW1.

Tonight's an Ativan and Milly night. G'night all.
[CA: Milly is my cat.]

3/15/20—password-protected journal, visible only to certain close friends

... my brother in Texas called me a snowflake this morning and sent me a photo of his MAGA hat. I had to send articles to my parents tonight to explain social distancing.

I only used one mask all day long. All 12 hours, although I really tried not to be in the room that much. The patient had come from a nursing home that we get a lot of patients from, and I've actually had them before. I don't think they really have it, but if they do, Jesus, everyone back at their home's a goner. They were already winning the Most Likely to Host a Pandemic race before this, they're a low-rent institution.

We intubated a 50-yr-old patient down the hall. They've got it. We don't know it for test-sure yet, but they're flu negative and they check all the other boxes.

Our higher-ups mandated no visitors at the hospital except for end-of-life reasons—our CEO came by to tell this to the visitors that we had and to help escort them out. This is great, because last night my patient's elderly spouse came in, in the rain on a freaking bus, and then chased me around the room trying to talk to me while I kept trying to stay the hell away.

They are now releasing expired masks for us to use.

Tomorrow's going to be interesting, as all the schools are closed and some of my coworkers aren't sure what they're going to do yet for childcare.

3/15/20

A coworker's husband, a respiratory therapist at another nearby facility, says they're already reusing their disposable blue gowns.

If supplies are this short now, we're going to be super hosed shortly.

3/18/20

I only used one mask this shift. I now have two extra. (All nurses are naturally kleptos (shut up, it's true).)

I'm trying to decide if I should pass these along or save them for when things get even more dire.

[CA: this was when our mask ration was 3 masks per shift.]

The shortage of face masks is so severe that the CDC is now advising nurses and other health care providers that they can "use homemade masks" like a "bandana" or "scarf" "as a last resort"—even though it admits the effectiveness "is unknown." (3/18/20)

3/18/20

If I have to start wearing a bandana to protect myself at work, I will embroider it with FUCK TRUMP first.

3/19/2020—password-protected journal

My mother finally has a friend whose kid has it. So while my parents have been good (or so they claim) about staying at home, now I know they really will be.

As for everything else—I have a few days off here. The calm before the storm. Been unable to concentrate on anything really, although I have book edits I need to do. (I did binge read a novel last night though, so that's something good.)

All the nurses in other countries are all wrapped up. In bunny suits, in practically Ebola gear.

And we're just... not.

We're on mask rations and going into rooms with skin still exposed because that's not normally a worrisome thing... until you see photos of nurses from Italy and China who're all heavily geared up, no skin at all visible. And now they're saying that health care workers who get it are more likely to die from it....

It doesn't feel good. I'm actually pretty scared. And y'all know me, I'm usually the person running into the spinning knives with abandon, heh.

I don't mind mitigated risk situations. I don't mind being

slightly more in danger. I'm stoic as fuck, and I've seen shit you wouldn't believe (and not just in a *Blade Runner* sense). But I don't want to feel like my time and efforts are being wasted, you know? I don't want to be thrown into a meat grinder because this country doesn't know the difference between its ass and a hole in the ground.

So yeah. That's where I'm at.

I had a two Ativan day the other day, one when I got home, and another so I could sleep four hours later because the first one didn't touch me. That's kind-of how panicky I am.

And I think I may have another now, and just take a blissful three-hour nap where I'm not worried about my next shift or my coworkers.

This feels a lot like being drafted for a war that some people still don't even believe we're in.

Present Day Thoughts

I don't think there's a way I can encapsulate the horror of knowing we were running out of supplies for you, the way every nurse across America lived it.

I have written 30+ books in my lifetime, and my metaphors still run dry. I can make attempts, but that is truly all they are.

It was like being a firefighter and told to go into a burning building without gear on.

Or being a teacher, teaching in one room, while there was an active shooter down the hall.

Or perhaps like going to war, knowing you didn't have enough body-armor on to protect yourself from bullets.

Here's where all those metaphors fail though—*they're time delineated.*

Firefighters do not spend 100% of their time running into fires.

The threat of an active shooter on campus, while utterly horrible and tragic, is usually limited to just one day. And even in a war, a soldier has downtime, traveling from base to base, or hiding between bursts of frenetic activity.

And?

In most of those circumstances?

The government—mostly—has your back. (Please don't get pedantic with me right now. I hate the NRA as much as you do; I realize how they've gutted our ability to do systemic gun violence studies, and I fucking hate that whole, "Stop the Bleed!" class that teenagers are given, so that they can, what, fucking pretend to be battlefield medics because we as a country cannot be bothered to protect them? Trust that I loathe hypocrisy in all its forms.)

But let me hop back a bit, first.

Do you release how frequently and aggressively nurses are audited? Some hospitals have entire managers who wander around looking at how your room is stocked. Not enough towels in the linen drawer? What else on earth could you have been doing!

I'm sure you don't believe it though, so let me prove it to you— you can close this book briefly now if you promise me you'll come back—go Google "nurse," "memes," and "whiteboard."

See how many memes there are that nurses have made because management has gotten mad at them for not "updating their whiteboard"?

Like writing down what day it is on a busy day is more important than saving lives?

I know it makes people happy when they see their nurse's name written up there, and I sure do like to write my patient's care goals up there—IF I FUCKING HAVE FREE TIME TO DO SO.

My hospital's pretty great about understanding this, actually, but I know from friends that there are skads of hospitals that aren't, who just have middle management roaming around like sleepless sharks looking for reasons to write you up, all the better to pretend they're doing something useful and you're not worthy of a raise.

I mention this because I want you to understand that, by and large, we're watched like hawks. And to some degree—issues with whiteboards notwithstanding—this makes sense, right? We're taking care of sick and helpless people. We have access to narcotics. We're expected to step up and accept accountability for our actions at every level.

So, while I can't speak for every state and every hospital, I want you to know this—in California, there are some offenses that are so outside the realm of acceptable patient care that, were you to be witnessed doing them, you would be assumed to be a danger to your patients and fired outright.

Do you know pre-covid, what one of these offenses would be?

Reusing isolation gear.

Imagine, your entire nursing career, you play by all these rules—don't recap needles, make sure you waste any unused narcotics or pharmacy will drop on your head, and if we catch you re-using a cheap plastic gown, we'll assume you're an idiot and you'll be written up or even fired (if we don't like you and you live in an at-will state without union protection).

And then, within the space of a goddamned week—week-and-a-half?—we were supposed to be okay with that?

Really?

Do the rules mean anything, or not?

Have we been living in isolation theater *our entire careers?*

Or, was it what felt more likely—*that the government did not care if we died?*

3/19/20

Can't stop thinking about how other countries are wrapping up their nurses practically head to toe and we're just not...or can't.

Can't stop thinking about my friends at work today.

3/19/20

All things considered, Ozymandias, I would've preferred another squid.

3/21/20—Text from a close friend at my prior job:

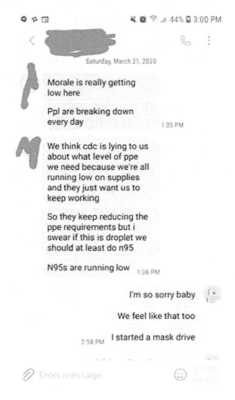

SO WE STARTED MASK-DRIVES.

Because in addition to saving lives, in addition to the stress of working at a hospital during a pandemic, it was important to get out there and do social networking TO TRY NOT TO FUCKING DIE.

I was going to write "I'm sorry if I sound pissed"—but, no, I'm not going to.

We were told to go out there and scrounge for our own protection.

LET ME REPEAT THAT: WE WERE TOLD TO GO OUT THERE AND SCROUNGE FOR OUR OWN PROTECTION.

CAN you even begin to imagine how fucked this was? How it felt?

It might've been different at the end of a war or something—supplies are low, everyone has to ration for the effort, after there's some coordinated national attempt that makes sense—but no, this was RIGHT AT THE FUCKING BEGINNING.

The first hospital I'd worked at wound up being one of the centers of covid for the Bay Area. They got hit. Hard.

And no one at the federal level cared.

Now, imagine being a person who knows that getting masks wet makes them unusable and unsafe.

Then imagine hearing Donald Trump, lamenting the "throwing away of the mask," because they can be "sanitized and reused," and claiming that "we have very good liquids for doing this," when you know very well no such thing exists.

Does it kill your soul quite as much as it killed mine?

3/21/20

Pretending to watch *Doctor Sleep* while madly tweeting people who say they can get masks to protect my beloved old coworkers and unsuccessfully trying not to cry, and tonight's going to be another Ativan night, dammit.

3/21/20

It's a good thing being a Millennial has been all about learning how to side hustle, seeing as right now my side hustle is finding people PPE so they can stay alive.

3/21/2020—personal journal

Lovely people have been donating masks on my doorstep (and others') and Trump this morning was on TV saying, and I quote, that we can just "wash masks."

That was the final straw for me. I screenshot it, sent it to my brother, and said, "Really?" and he called and said Trump was misquoted (he wasn't) and that "all this is going to blow over," etc.

So I told him I was accepting donations of masks at my house because we're on rations now, and he still didn't care—but he is a firefighter. So I asked him how he'd feel going into a burning building without his gear on.

He said it "wasn't comparable" and "if I didn't want to do my job I should quit it."

I told him I'd talk to him in a month and hung up.

I know my brother loves Trump. I knew that before this and I don't even know why I thought this would change things. My husband is in possession of my phone now, so that I don't do anything bad with it. I'm trying to figure out if I should puke, cry, or take Ativan.

They've started offering overtime at work. My husband doesn't want me to go in before my next shift, Tues, because right now we're both safe and healthy and we should enjoy that. I feel selfish, but he's also right. This is going to be a marathon.

3/22/20

I got a line on some masks, and I now have a sudden appreciation for how it must've felt to be a coke dealer in the '80s.

Yo, man, you know where I can score some n95s?

3/22/2020—personal journal

Late-night hustling—I found a lawyer at Microsoft who's arranging bulk mask purchases from China AND a lawyer from Rutgers who used to work for the Clinton Foundation in China and has access to masks, and coordinated getting them in touch with my old hospital this morning. [CA: I never got the chance to follow up and see if these donations made it through, but I did CC these people and my old boss to put them in touch.]

It made all my Twitter trolling feel very, very worthwhile, phew.

And a friend dropped masks off on my porch this morning! :D

The burden feels a little lighter today <3

3/23/2020

My parents just drove five hrs. round trip to drop off six n95 masks and homemade caramel corn in my laundry room. We said hi, we couldn't hug, and I got to show them a little of my backyard at a safe distance, if anyone wants to note the time and date of when all this shit broke me.

California is looking for 595 million masks and a billion gloves, according to Newsom. Goddamn.

The Lt Gov of Texas says on TV that "grandparents would be happy to die for their children." (3/23/20)

AND, also, around this time last March was when childish libertarian-slash-state's-responsibilities assholes rose up from the ground like so many supply-side Lazaruses, talking shit about how hospitals should've had enough material for this in stock, like they've ever worked in materials management before.

A major hospital in NYC goes through a million masks a week—just masks! Not even gowns, or gloves!—in *normal* circumstances.

Covid-times were not normal times.

There would've been no possible way for any single facility to be prepared for covid at one institution, much less at all institutions in a hospital system—or across a state!—simultaneously.

The reason no hospital was sitting on a month's worth of isolation supplies at any one time, ahead of time, hoarding them like Smaug's gold, was this: Where the fuck would you store it all?

There likely aren't even a million blades of grass in your frontyard, libertarian-sir.

You don't own a million of shit.

So how the fuck was every hospital in America supposed to have locked in 2-3 months of supplies, Suzie-fucking-Ormand emergency-style, just in case, for a ONCE-IN-A-LIFETIME EMERGENCY?

This was why we *needed the federal government to take charge.*

Desperately.

But it wouldn't, because Trump and the GOP couldn't profit off of competence... and then stuff like this started to happen: Larry Kudlow, Trump's top economic advisor on FOX news said, "The president is right. The cure can't be worse than the disease. And we're going to have to make some difficult tradeoffs."

"The cure"—by which he meant the methods we might use to save lives, like going into total lockdown with adequate universal basic income to make it so that everyone could afford to eat and pay rent while they're staying safe, and encouraging widespread mask use....

"...than the disease"—by which he means the virus that will go on to claim six hundred thousand lives.

They could not be bothered to save lives.

THEY COULD NOT BE BOTHERED TO SAVE LIVES.

The GOP would rather piss on the ashes of six hundred thousand people than lift a reasonable finger to do anything to stop them from being harmed.

If that doesn't tell you all you need to know about the GOP, well, I don't know what to say. (I know I'm preaching to the choir here, most likely. But sometimes it's good to hear someone else say what you're thinking. It helps you to triangulate yourself.)

And before you get all, "Well, it was only the elderly," go fuck yourself. "It was only the black or brown people." Go fuck yourself. "Only the fat people." Go fuck yourself. Or "Only the people with diabetes"? You can go fuck yourself, too.

What kind of miserable trash human are you, to decide that someone else's life is not worth living?

Who appointed you God-king of life and death?

Fuck, man, I'm the one sitting at the bedside at the end with the morphine, and even *I* don't feel that fucking power.

What the fuck is wrong with them?

THIS IS a great time for a segue, since I'm on the topic.

Who the fuck do you think watched six hundred thousand people die in the United States so far? Because I bet you no more than a few thousand of those people managed to make it home to die, with hospice or without, since we would never send someone home with active covid to infect the rest of their family.

But let's pretend maybe a hundred thousand got out—fine, that still leaves us with half a million corpses.

Who held their hands, or tried to, through gloves? Who held phones and iPads up so that they could hear your last words and maybe see your face one last time? Who took care of them for hours, days, weeks, months, greeting you on the phone by name, until your loved one's final passing?

Who tried to give them dignity, in a place and time where it was sorely lacking? Who tried to show them the compassion when portions of the outside world were saying that covid—the very thing that was clotting their blood and stealing their breath—was a lie?

It was *us*. The nurses.

It was only goddamned March, we were hip deep in the first wave, and the government's already asking us to go into battle without gear on and talking about *acceptable casualties*.

I think I finally found my metaphor.

Nursing then was like being asked to save lives on a sinking ship, knowing that you and everyone aboard was going to drown.

3/23/20

Zolpidem Tartrate take me awayyyyyyyyyyy.
    [CA: Ambien is the brand name.]

Trump wants to end the shut down on Easter because it'd be "beautiful" to have churches packed all across the nation. (3/24/20)

3/24/2020—personal journal

Had two suspected cases this morning. Around 9, there was a gaggle of RNs outside, getting news from our charge nurse, and one looked at me (in a suspected patient's room), made a plus sign with her fingers, and jerked her chin next door.

He was the one we thought would be positive—he had a super fever, and the "ground glass" look in his lungs on scans.

I hadn't gone into his room by then. We were trialing this whole "pumps outside the room with extension IV tubing" deal, so there was no reason to go in (even with a suspected patient) until I had to, seeing as we were trying to keep contact to a minimum (which, it turns out, we can't do, because we'll run out of tubing too fast, so real exciting trial there).

As you might imagine, going into that room for the first time, knowing what we all know now, sucked.

Especially knowing that I'd been rationed one (1!) mask for the day.

But—things got better. He was an easy patient. He's getting better, despite being on the vent. I grouped my tasks. I made sure respiratory didn't have to go in. I waited and went in again with nightshift when they came on board, so that no one else had to risk themselves, seeing as she and I were already risking it, and that way we didn't have to drag in others. I usually run a tight ship anyhow. I hate it when break RNs have to do stuff for me, so that was just like normal.

It was good to be around my coworkers and see some other

humans. It was good to feel our collective worry together and not feel like it's just me on the couch all the time.

It was just good to be working, really. I'm like a sled dog; I'm always happiest in a harness, pulling.

I got to hear about our contingency plans. There's plans to kick our ICU up to 50 beds if we need to, taking over PACU and OR. Even possibly taking over step-down (the next level care down from ICU) and pushing them to some other floor. They've also gotten 19 step-down nurses to volunteer to be trained, so they're starting to shadow us ASAP.

Newsom has lifted title 22, which is the ratio law in CA, so from here on out there are no RN to patient ratios (which makes sense, considering). If shit gets real, we can give these step-down RNs some stable patients, ones who don't need vent changes or drip titration, and we can take the harder ones—because opening up 2x as many beds doesn't automatically mean magically having staff for all of them.

Tomorrow I'm going to go run errands and drop off the masks people have been sending me and see if (God, please God) the Starbucks in the Safeway is open while I get some prescriptions filled.

Not back on till Friday <3.

3/24/20

For years I've winced as families watched Fox news in the rooms of their sick/dying elders, not understanding that Trump would put their loved one on an ice floe and personally kick them out to sea.

Well, here we are.

At least now I'm the only person in charge of the channel.

3/24/20

If I keep taking showers that hot, I'm going to find out what my real hair color is in T minus three weeks here.

3/24/20

You might have noticed that I've stopped pleading for PPEs. It isn't because we don't still need them; we do. But I'm only taking them from local people now, because I'd feel like a jerk stealing them from some other state. We're all on the same ride now, acknowledged or not.

ON 3/25, frustrated by the President's apparent inability to understand why NYC needed ventilators so badly, I did my first viral tweet about lungs, oxygenation, and how ventilators work. I later wrote an essay on the topic for my author's newsletter, a place where I generally try to stay chirpy because I'd like the people reading it to buy my fiction.

If you'd like to read a 2,000-word essay on lung function for your edification, here you go—but if you don't want to science-nerd so hard, feel free to skip past.

The TL;DR version is this: lungs are important, and Trump was evil.

TODAY I'M GOING to explain oxygenation and ventilation in layman's terms, so y'all can play the home game!

People on the internet have been throwing around terms like ventilators, non-invasive ventilators, respirators, modified snorkles, 3D-printed things, and sharing hacks where you can run four people off of the same ventilator. My intention here is to help break that down so that everyone can understand what we mean when we talk about those terms and why ventilation is so important, particularly in covid cases.

Let's begin at the beginning—what is oxygen and why do you need it? The oxygen in the air you breathe is part of the Krebs cycle, which is a biochemical process that produces ATP, the building block of energy for your body. Your body gets the oxygen it needs out of your lungs. When you drown, your lungs are filled with water, and this oxygen transfer can't occur. No ATP equals death. (Randomly, because if you're reading this far, we're all nerds—the reason cyanide kills you is it blocks another function in the Krebs cycle, which also = no ATP = death.)

So! There are several different levels of oxygenating people. We'll go from lightest to strongest.

The first is a nasal canula—you've seen these on TV. They've got the two prongs that fit into your nose (which don't create a perfect seal; we'll come back to that in a bit here)—they basically goose your lungs with a little extra oxygen.

If that's not enough, we can move through a series of more intense face masks till we get to a non-rebreather. You've probably seen these on TV, too; they're the cone-mask looking ones with the inflatable air bags behind them, like you see on the drawings of "in case of loss of pressure" on an airplane. These have a better seal (to keep that oxygen in!) and can provide 100% oxygen.

We usually only use non-rebreathers during an emergency. If you're in a situation where you need 100% oxygen, you are doing very poorly. Atmospheric oxygen concentrations are 21%, so you can see that us giving you 100% oxygen is a lot more than that. It's also a bad idea to blast people with 100% oxygen for too long, as it represses your respiratory drive to breathe.

If a 100% rebreather's not cutting it—there's two possible reasons why:

1. Your airway is blocked. You could be drunk, passed out, a stroke victim, choking, or have apnea—at this stage we say you're "not protecting your airway." This makes sense because, if the oxygen isn't getting into your lungs, it means there's a blockage somewhere, right?
2. Your airway is fine, but your lungs are damaged.

YOUR LUNGS ARE tissue-paper-thin organs that inflate and deflate a kajillion times over the course of your life. Over time, they lose elasticity and compliance, especially as you age. You can go to the gym all you want to, but you can't really keep your lungs "youthful" indefinitely.

The functional unit of your lungs are an air sacs called an alveoli. They're lined with a surfactant that keeps them open and inflatable, otherwise their walls would stick together after they collapsed. (It's the lack of this surfactant before a certain gestational week that makes life so difficult for preemies.) Inside your alveoli is where the magic happens—because the entire job of your lungs is to serve as the intersection between the outside world's oxygen and your internal body's blood supply.

Your alveoli are wrapped in miles of tiny capillaries, tissue against tissue, and that's where this oxygen transfer occurs. You breathe in your normally 21% oxygenated air in normal life, your alveoli inflate, and the tension of that inflation helps to stick the lung tissue to the capillary network surrounding them.

This is when and where that oxygen jumps from the air into your blood supply, to be whisked around and used to eventually make energy.

Does that make sense? I hope so! Have I almost typed ravioli twenty times already? Yes.

So! You need air to live! How's it going to get in there if you can't breathe?

Sometimes just adding pressure helps. You probably know all about this because of a relative's CPAP machine. That's what we call 'Non-Invasive Ventilation'—because we're not using an "invasive breathing tube." The CPAP machine creates a seal around a person's face—important to keep air in!—and shoves that normal 21% atmospheric oxygen in there to help get around whatever's blocking your airway.

These are nice to use in the hospital if you can, because intubating someone is highly invasive. However, with covid patients, CPAP and their cousin BiPAP machines are dangerous because they've got exhalation valves that essentially (we think) aerosolize the covid and spray it out everywhere. So the patient's better off—because yay breathing! But the health care workers helping them in their rooms have to be extra careful.

But sometimes people's lungs need higher concentrations of oxygen, due to damage, age, pre-existing conditions like COPD, or they can't protect their airways because they're so exhausted from trying to breathe, or they're passed out, etc.

That's when we intubate you.

Intubation is when they put a breathing tube through your mouth down to where your lungs branch off right and left. How do we keep that air in there? Great question! There's an inflatable ring around the tube that we inflate once the tube is in position, allowing us to keep the higher concentrations of oxygen you need in there without leaking and allowing us to give you oxygen at higher pressures to keep your lungs inflated.

Okay, you're tubed—now what?

Now, we put that tube to a ventilator. A ventilator is a machine that is capable of managing all sorts of factors that go into breathing for you, according to what the doctors think will be most therapeutic for your lungs. (Respiratory therapists are some of the most unsung heroes during all of this—they're going into rooms to assess and make changes all the time; they work hand in hand with RNs and MDs to make sure you get your air.)

The most important things a ventilator can do are:

1. Control your percent of oxygenation. The more you need, the worse off you are, alas.
2. Control the number of breaths you take, sometimes with the help of sedation.
3. Control the pressure (or force) with which you receive your oxygen. This is called PEEP, which stands for positive end expiratory pressure. A normal PEEP is 5. A drowning victim's PEEP setting might be as high as 20, because you're trying to shove air in there through all that water.
4. Control the volume of oxygen that you're given, measured in mLs.

OUR IMAGINARY PATIENT was sedated prior to getting intubated and temporarily paralyzed so they won't fight tube insertion. Getting a breathing tube put in you and then having to breathe through that tube, which I've heard is like breathing through a straw, is almost universally upsetting, so we typically keep people on a little sedation after the tube is in, just so they won't be freaked out or remember things as clearly.

When you get sick from covid, a lot of things can happen to your body, but one of the worst of them is this: ARDS. It stands for Acute Respiratory Distress Syndrome.

ARDS is hard to survive under the best conditions. It's got

wicked mortality rates that only increase as you get older and lose that lung elasticity/compliance, as I mentioned before.

ARDS gets you a couple different ways—due to inflammation on a cellular level, the surfactant layers inside your alveoli break down so you can't transfer oxygen across to your capillaries. Your alveoli fill up with mucus, so you can't transport oxygen. And the final kicker is that that inflammation also causes the interstitial space between where your alveoli and your capillaries should touch to widen—also preventing oxygen transfer.

How a ventilator helps is this: We can give you a higher concentration of oxygen (while remembering that riding straight 100% for too long is bad). We can help you to breathe more effectively by controlling your breaths, using sedation. We can increase the pressure with which you receive your oxygen, helping to keep what functional alveoli you have working, and we can control the volume of oxygen we given you, both to keep the alveoli inflated.

SOMETIMES WE WILL EVEN PARALYZE and "prone" you, to make use of the larger lung-tissue surface area at your back. Paralyzing you lets us take your lungs "offline" so that the ventilator does their job for them. We don't want you wasting any precious energy—literally precious, because oxygen equals energy, remember?—on the work of breathing.

Our goal is to use the ventilator's settings, giving you the greatest chance at survival by keeping the functional parts of your lungs working, if we can. But everything has its limits, alas.

We can't over-inflate your lungs with too much pressure, they'll pop. We can't give you too much volume, see popping. 100% oxygenation can be bad long term, and it doesn't matter how many breaths we give you if your lung tissue just isn't able to do its job, you know?

So—if you've come this far with me, you are in for the full science ride, but content warning: death ahead—why are all those people in New York dying? Because, like I said, ARDS is extremely dangerous under optimal conditions. How do you die of ARDS? Basically, you wind down due to lack of oxygen, because you can't make ATP. And internally, you drown.

And this is why when people say, "Oh, we can just attach four people to one vent!" I kind-of want to hurt someone. Yes, it's been done under trauma conditions, most notably the Vegas shooting not that long ago, but the pressure, volume, and percent oxygen needs for your 95 lb. grandma versus a 250 lb. college kid are vastly different, which should make sense to y'all now, right?

Also? I'd just really rather not be in battle triage scenarios if timely creation or purchasing and sending of equipment can help.

3/27/20

Every morning when I wake up, my jaw is tight enough to bite through submarine steel.

3/28/20

We're out of disposable gowns now. Materials management came by to try to restock us with sterile gowns instead.

My two isolation carts still have enough to make it through my shift, but dang.

So now, because we're short on gowns, I shouldn't even go into my patient's rooms if I wanted to.

I hate this new normal.

4/1/20

Just wanted to show you all what the local Boy Scouts made
for us to use at work:

    [CA: a photo of a homemade face shield was attached to
this tweet]

4/1/20

Astrology for April:
    Aquarius: stay the fuck inside
    Pisces: stay the fuck inside
    Cancer: stay the fuck inside
    Aries: stay the fuck inside
    Taurus: stay the fuck inside
    Virgo: stay the fuck inside
    Libra: stay the fuck inside
    Sagittarius: stay the fuck inside

Scorpio: stay the fuck inside

This series of tweets was made on 4/1/20 in response to the "You signed up for this!" argument, wherein people tried to claim that by virtue of having signed up to be nurses, we'd become contractually obligated to go on suicide missions without adequate PPE.

I want to talk about the level of things I've signed onto by being a nurse, too, so people don't just think we're crying wolf. I have:

Been kicked.

Been punched (at, none landed).

Had a patient attempt to bite me.

Been on a campus with a gunman.

Been covered in blood.

Been splashed in the eye with blood.

Been stuck by a dirty needle.

Have had to clean up more blood, vomit, shit.

Have had to deal with dangerously aggressive patients & family members.

Have had to know where my exits are.

Have flirted my way out of trouble before. Not sexy-times flirting, but the whole "oh come on now, I'm just a girl" thing you do around abusers to get clear.

Have had patients threaten to come back and shoot all of us with the guns you knew they actually had.

Took care of a patient whose gangster boyfriend had

already burned her car and house, and splashed her with acid, so the willingness to escalate was pretty much there.

This is all on top of what I used to do as a burn nurse, which was pretty much peeling at people's skin.

And you know what, I am so, so, so, so, so not alone. Like, we're already putting ourselves in danger every single time we go to work. There's a reason we have mandated "workplace violence protection" classes every year.

So when people tell us that we should suck it up, as though we have not sucked it up already and have been sucking it up for decades because it's our dang job and we want to draw one—one!—reasonable line in the sand for PPE —it pisses me off.

PS: I forgot all the times I've been spit at and yelled at. So much yelling.

Oh, the joys of nursing....

4/1/20

If only hubris cured coronavirus.

Trump says, "We're a backup, we're not an ordering clerk," in regard to state-vs-state competition for PPE and supplies. When asked what happens when states compete, he says, "They have that, and they have to work that out." (4/2/20)

4/2/20

They're going to start doing temps on us when we come into work tomorrow.

My coworker: "It's rectal. Bring your own lube."

4/3/2020—personal journal

We went from three cases to nine cases today. Just in my ICU.

They divided my ICU into one wing covid, one wing non-covid, and our AMAZING engineers made the covid side negative pressure, which is awesome.

The downside is that they kept sending people who they thought didn't have covid to my side, where we weren't wearing N95 masks, just surgical droplet ones.

We had one patient who had had surgery on their extremity. Their surgical site got infected, and they stayed home because they were afraid of coming to the hospital and getting covid....

Whelp, they came to our side, went into respiratory failure, wound up intubated, and their CT scan came back positive (via radiology) before their covid-test came back. So they already had it, but now they've got it plus necrotizing fasciitis.

And we got another patient who was in a car accident, who spiked up to 103.5—turns out they'd just returned from a trip to NYC, which we didn't know about because they couldn't talk when they were brought in....

So yeah.

We wound up moving them over to the official covid wing, but getting yelled at halfway thru the shift to put PPE on was thrilling (not).

Hilariously, for some values thereof, surgery ran through after hearing about their infected patient and they were freaking out about having done surgery on him without proper protection, and we were all, "Welcome to the front lines."

Anyhow.

Shit's real. Realer.

Also, the on-call they were offering earlier—prior to today, they could cancel us for it. Now, they say if we're on call we get paid no matter what.

Because they need us. It's about to hit the fan.

4/3/20

Our intensivist just came up from seeing possible admits in the ED. "I hate to say it, but I think our surge is here."

4/3/20

I'll tell you what, now is a really bad time to have an anxiety disorder.

4/4/20—password protected journal

Hey also—I've been thinking about [redacted's] last paragraph all night.

I don't know who needs to hear this, but—I want to hear all y'alls things.

I know sometimes I come into here hot (especially after a shift) and I am in a mood (especially after a shift) and y'all know I have a temper.

BUT.

I want to hear all y'alls things.

I don't want anyone ever to think they can't share whatever's happening to them here because it's not "enough." I don't want to suck up the oxygen in this thread. There's no competition here for any of our assorted pains to feel valid. We're all stuck together on a trip that none of us wanted to be on. I may be nearer the boiler room, but the ship is still going down with all of us aboard.

What's more, is I *need* to hear your things.

After I started in burn I got this peculiar kind of PTSD (undiagnosed, but highly likely) and like—it's hard to reintegrate into society. It makes me shit at parties, as I can generally only tell sad stories about serious things. You start feeling like you're different, even though you know you're not, and it is not good. Sometimes you feel megalomaniacal-different, because you want to psych yourself up and pretend that your sacrifice has more meaning than it does, sometimes it's ostracized-from-society-different because no one else understands you at all.

I can feel it happening again to me now. I don't want it to. So I just want to check in and make sure that everyone feels good about posting here/there/everywhere right now.

I treat all of y'alls posts here and in all the other threads like wartime letters from home. I enjoy knowing what's going on with everyone else. I enjoy feeling interconnected. I remember our shared past so fondly. I have such hopes for our collective futures.

So, yeah. Please, everyone, carry on. Don't be embarrassed about sharing bad news or good news or just popping in to say that you're still OK. I want to know everything; really, I do. I don't care if you post forty times a day, if that's what you need and it's good for your mental well-being. This is me, absolving everyone utterly of any hesitation, okay?

We've never needed each other more than in this moment.

I love y'all.

THIS WAS my next viral Twitter thread on 4/4/20, about end-of-life decision making.

Okay, I have passed from incandescent rage stage to just wanting to explain things calmly, so I'll post:

Hello, I would like to tell you what it's like to put your loved one to sleep from the medical side. This might be a long thread. Buckle in.

In a perfect world, this would be a decision the patient would participate in themselves.

This should now be a legit discussion you have with your family members.

If you don't let people know what your desires are—well, they won't know. And they'll hesitate.

No one wants to be the bad guy who pulls the plug. And without clear guidance from you, your family is going to feel guilty. No matter what they decide.

So please, please, please, have those talks. Even though they're scary. They're important.

Onwards:

Once it's decided, via your decision, prior discussion with your family, the existence of a POLST (a document where you delineate what kind of medical care is acceptable to you), or at the bedside as your condition deteriorates....

The doctors will write the orders for "comfort care" and/or "compassionate extubation."

If you're not intubated (i.e., not on a ventilator) then they'll probably downgrade your care to a lower-level floor, where the nurses will be able to give you medications to help control your pain.

They'll turn off the monitors and do whatever they can to keep you "comfortable" at that time. That might be feeding you regular food, even if you can't properly swallow or if it's a choice between eating and not breathing—because if you're with it enough to want a brownie, we're going try to let you eat one.

Most people just take a few bites or sips of water and relax.

From our side of the bed, those pleasures seem fleeting, but intense.

And, essentially, we'll let you wind down, giving you narcotics along the way.

Let's hop back to the people who were intubated, though, and chase that half of the flowchart down.

In those cases, we arrange a time with respiratory to remove the tube. Hopefully, family is there.

Usually the doctors give us orders for a solid push of morphine to start. 10 mgs or so?

No one wants to see you "air hungry." That's what it is. When you can't get enough air in. It's horrific to watch and I am certain it is horrific to experience.

The respiratory therapist will deflate the cuff holding your breathing tube in and take it out of your throat. Your throat will be sore.

Hopefully, the push of prior meds was enough to make you "comfortable." We oftentimes hook people up to morphine drips at this point to give them additional pain control, or we commit ourselves to checking on you very regularly, with additional pushes of morphine in our pockets —sometimes we just get a ton out of the medication machine and return what we didn't use later. 2-4 mgs every 2-5 mins, depending on the orders.

No one's going to refuse you/us more orders at that point, either. Because no one wants to watch you suffer. I once dumped 40 mgs into an adult man in what let's just say was a "quick" amount of time, because it was that or have everyone stare in horror as he couldn't breathe....

What I'm saying is that things can be liberal if need be.

It doesn't always go quickly, though. Sometimes people can manage slowly on their own for days, usually getting downgraded like our brownie-eating friend.

The monitor in the room is definitely off, but we can still see things at the nursing station. So we know what your numbers are, and when your heart starts to slow.

We can give you robinul, which stops you from salivating

so much, so it doesn't sound traumatic and harsh to whoever's watching....

Our goal really is to just make you "comfortable" without pushing you over the edge too quickly. That's what divides it from actual euthanasia, I suppose. It's not planned. It can sometimes take longer than you think.

I always try to prepare families for that.

Once people make the decision about their loved one, they always feel like it's jumping off a cliff—and they rather think that pulling out a breathing tube is like flipping off a light switch. It's not always. Like I said, sometimes things can take days.

My goal, bedside, is to try to honor you somehow. To make sure that someone's watching when you go. To hopefully doula your family through that horrified stage where they're all staring at your slowing breathing, and over to the story-telling time part.

Once people start laughing because of the stories they're telling inside a comfort care room, I know things are going to be okay.

Losing you is still going to hurt them, but they'll remember you, you know?

I don't know yet, personally, how covid is going change all that. We're on the upswing of our wave at my facility, so it is hard to imagine.

And there are some people who never accept death or dying, who are angry at the world until the end.

And I've seen some clearly tortured elderly patients whose families couldn't let them go. I swear I am not a eugenicist—but man, people just don't get to live forever. You start breaking down, your lungs, kidneys, hearts, skin. You give out.

The American relationship with death and dying is pretty

fucked. And I know no one wants their loved ones to die. But sometimes we just don't get that choice, you know?

Anyhow.

I have no idea how to end this, honestly. I don't want to scare you about what's coming.

But at the same time I would feel like a jerk if I didn't at least try to educate in some small way whenever and wherever I could.

Every time I comfort care someone, I feel in some small way like I'm killing them. Even if it's not true.

I hate it. And I hate that I'm good at it. Because I'm some sort of weird empathy sponge and families need me.

I buy plants every time I comfort care a patient. I work in a ward with a lot of elderly people.

I have a very, very nice garden.

So I guess I'll end with this—please stay indoors.

All of this shit is going to be horrific enough. I don't want to watch people die if I don't have to. I don't want you to not be there to see it.

No one is going to be there to laugh with me.

I won't know their stories.

I won't really be able to make them feel less alone. And each time I do my job, a little piece of my soul dies.

(My close friends know how close I was to quitting before all this, and this is why.)

And that's all. Sorry I got wandery; I started off strong and then I started crying, so here we are.

Just stay inside. Please.

Don't make me work harder than I have to.

4/7/20

Today's patient is not doing well.

Their lungs are leaking air, AKA crepitus. It's trapped underneath their skin on their chest. If you listen to it as you touch it, it sounds like Rice Krispies popping gently as you break the air bubbles and they reform.

4/7/20

Saw a bunch of feet beneath the curtain outside my covid patient's room. Management.

I assume I'm in trouble, of course. I was born with a guilty conscience, for what I don't know.

No.

They're counting gowns housewide. Because we're going to run out.

Hospitals say feds are seizing masks and other coronavirus supplies without saying a word. (4/7/20)

4/7/20

Drove home at 85 mph on an empty highway with the windows down and "Glorious" by MUSE cranked so I could feel alive.

Then I turned it down when I got into my neighborhood because I'm not an animal, and started crying.

4/8/20—excerpt from my author newsletter

...I had a nice weekend off and then I spent the past two days on the covid side with two covid patients. One old, one younger than me. The old one is definitely going to pass; they just don't have the biological reserves left to fight. Like I talked about in my ventilator post last time, your lungs just don't stay the same over time, you know?

The person younger than me—that was tough. They were younger than my little brother. In the prime of their life, in all other respects.

We've got this patient on the drugs the President is touting [CA: HCQ—hydroxychloroquine]—because their heart can handle it. That's the unfortunate thing with Trump shouting from the rooftops about that certain drug combination. Regardless of the facts of whether it winds up working (and recent studies from France say, no, not really) the drugs he's hyping can be very, very dangerous. I had this kid on the monitor setting so I can watch not only his heart rhythm all the time, like normal for the ICU, but also his QTc ratio. Your QTc ratio measures a portion of the electrical timing between one part of your heartbeat and another.

If you listen to someone else's heart, you've heard the lub-dub there, right? It's two separate phases. That's because electricity flows over your heart and triggers different parts of it at different times. Your upper chambers kind-of cock the gun, putting that blood into your lower chambers, and then your larger lower chambers shoot it up into your lungs to get it oxygenated or out into your body. All of that is a timed event though. And if you think about it you can understand why it'd be bad to have those chambers out of sync—if you can't load, you can't fire, right?

So the meds that the president keeps talking about have the ability to offset the timing between the chambers in your heart. And if those chambers get offset badly enough you will die.

That's why when you take them, you need to be closely monitored. If your timing gets wider, we can stop giving you those meds—

but it's also why you absolutely should not be taking them at home, unsupervised, and definitely not without having had at least an EKG first. My older patient? We couldn't give her those meds because it was unlikely her heart could take it. And there's a segment of the population out there who already have long-QT syndrome genetically and don't even know it! If they took those meds because their friendly whoever prescribed them for them thoughtlessly, they might die.

I know everyone wants a solid answer to this thing. I know everyone wants a miracle cure. I really want one too. But we're not there yet, alas, and it may be quite some time. The only reliably life-saving things we can do right now are stay inside as much as possible, limit our contacts with others, and wear masks and gloves in public spaces.

Overall, my facility is lucky—we're not getting hit as hard as some places I know, although we all do feel like our time is coming. But it is hard to feel lucky in a room where you're treating someone for something that doesn't have a reliable cure. I've taken care of TB people before (oh my gosh, I could inundate y'all with an arm's length of letter acronyms of Things I Have Treated In The Past: C. diff, VRE, CRE, MRSA, etc.) but this is very different, emotionally. It's a kind of existential dread, you know? It's always there. It's not going anywhere. It's endless. Like knowing that you're being chased by a steamroller and someone's gone and nailed down both your feet.

People keep telling us that we're heroes, which is sweet, but I didn't sign on to do this to be a hero. I just wanted a fun non-office job, and writing didn't pay the bills. (Getting to hang out with some of the most fantastic strong-willed women in the world, though, was an unexpected benefit. I treasure my nurse friends so, so much.) But I don't want to have to be a hero. I just want to do a good job, safely, and for all of my friends and patients to get to make it out of this alive. That's all I've ever wanted, really. And that's still what I want, for all of us.

Okay, phew. That's enough for today. I appreciate you reading this far, as always, and I always read responses and respond, even if it's just with a <3 [CA: a heart]. I don't want to smiley anyone so much anymore, because I don't want other people to think that I'm in any way happy that we're in this situation together. And I'm sorry my responses aren't always longer. I can't claim to have massive amounts of an attention span or bandwidth right now, I vacillate between wanting-to-cry, crying, and aftermath-of-crying pretty much daily.

But <3 means I'm thinking of you and thank you for thinking about me.

<3
Cassie

4/8/20—password protected journal

Last night was my lowest night yet.

That's kind of saying something, as many of my nights these past few weeks have been low.

I took care of two ppl with covid these past two days and the cognitive dissonance of doing what I do with one mask (and now they're talking about rationing disposable gowns) and then watching the president lie out his ass on TV, is intense. Like he's ever done one good thing this whole time. Fuck him in the neck forever.

And now I read today about how FEMA and the government are stealing supplies legitimately bought by states or overbidding smaller states, likely so they can give these supplies to their cronies and sell them back at absolutely usurious rates (see Maddow last night) and like—what the absolute clown fuck is going the hell on?

I have no choice but to think that all of the GOP, from the President on down, wants me to die.

Literally anyone who votes for him again is voting for me (and possibly everyone else! We all get to play the home game!) to die.

I posited this view this morning on the phone with my mother, who tried to blame the Chinese, and I pointed out that Trump's administration ignored Obama's pandemic instructions and defunded the CDC, and she told me those were my opinions and I said, no, truth is not opinions and hung up.

And science is goddamned science, and I will not hear the fuck otherwise ever again.

I knew that this, and all the other governmental erosion that's happened these past years, would be an inevitable consequence of living in a post-truth society. I had just hoped that we'd see the light in time, before something like this, and somehow steer the train back on the tracks.

But no. People had to be worried about imaginary immigration issues and imaginary voter fraud and imaginary infringement of religious rights. People forgot what the fuck empathy was and that the point of having a society was to LIVE IN IT and not hoard your resources and protect them at gunpoint.

People wanted something "different!" They "couldn't get excited about a woman."

And now I get to go to work and treat people who have contagious diseases for which there are no cure.

Table-fucking-flip.

I'm livid. And when I'm not livid I'm crying. And people on Twitter are calling nurse friends of mine crisis actors like that is EVEN A FUCKING THING, and there are those asshats who are promoting the "film your hospital" hashtag because they don't believe that we're in there working, and OTHER PEOPLE who are GODDAMNED ON RIGHT NOW are trying to say that if you have another disease and covid, then your covid death shouldn't count?

That's like saying if you have COPD, but you're in a car wreck, your car wreck shouldn't count towards car wreck numbers.

It's not a gotcha. It's just illustrating how mind-blowingly medically and mathematically illiterate you are. Not to mention fucking gullible as shit.

So yeah.

I'm incandescent.

I can't quit because people (namely my coworkers) need me. But I'm not excited about going into work. I'm not thrilled by taking the chance of getting a higher viral load and dying. I don't appreciate the US government trying to dick me over without lube.

And I swear to God that when this is over, should it end, I will never forgive the people who still stand behind him.

I might delete this in an hour or two when I'm less angry. If I'm less angry though it's because I am off crying.

I don't want to be tough and I don't want to be a hero and I don't want to die for bullshit reasons because a bullshit man has to pretend to run the country.

It didn't have to be like this.

A meme starts going around the internet, saying "Essential workers—because sacrificial sounded too dark." (4/8/20)

4/9/20

FML you guys.

Just went to the CT scanner with this patient.

This guy's lungs look like shit.

I haven't been wearing an n95 all day because we've been "conserving" them.

4/9/20

The ceremonial unmasking in my car is undoubtedly the best part of every shift now.

4/11/2020—password protected journal

...honestly, until we're all n95 everywhere (which we might never be) I'd almost rather be on the covid side of my floor one hundred percent of the time, where I'll have an n95 and know what's up, rather than not be given one and get caught with my guard down.

Shitty to have to think like that though.

Today, on the covid side, with two positive patients, I was given three plastic disposable gowns for an entire 12-hr shift.

record scratch

I cycled through the entire DABDA [CA: the traditional cycle of grief], wanting to puke/cry/cuss/yell, and then dug through all the shit in equipment rooms till I found two chemo gowns—the gowns we use when we give meds that are dangerous—and claimed them and reused them in the rooms I had, hanging them up inside of the room for me to put on once I was inside, repeatedly, until around noon, when someone from materials management coughed up a fresh box of gowns.

And then I kept using my gowns that I'd hustled because, shit, we're a twenty-four-hour operation, what the fuck's night shift going to use?

Mind you, the chemotherapy gowns I was using are also supposed to be disposable. They're just slightly nicer than normal gowns is all. Easier than flimsy plastic to keep in one piece.

Random Management Types came through today with the bright idea of putting the pumps closer to the doors so we can make pump changes without gowns on, which is great and all—but we tried using extension tubing for our pumps literally the first covid case I had, and our boss said back then we didn't have enough tubing to do that.

And one of my coworkers threw a shit-fit because in order to move the pumps close enough to the doors to work you have to move the bed closer, too—and if you're under 6 feet from the patient touching the pump without a gown on, what the fuck's the point?

Anyhow.

Who the fuck knows?

I am doing my damnedest to be safe, but honestly the longer this goes on, and I know it will be going on for a long, long time, the more obvious it is that me not catching it—or surviving it quickly/asymptomatically—will be a matter of luck and not anything else I do.

I'm not going to work in a room without a gown.

4/11/20

Hey Cassie, watcha doin'?

Oh, you know, just buying long-sleeve ponchos off of Amazon in case I need them for work because this is what it's like now. Lolsob.

4/12/20

WHERE'S YOUR NIHILISM NOW????

Oh. Over here. Right where I left it.

4/13/20

I wouldn't trust anyone on Trump's Reopen America taskforce to successfully open a jar of pickles.

4/13/20—personal journal

Every day I have off and out of the hospital I think about Doing A Thing and every day off I wind up in a funk of not doing anything, with the exception of about 30 clear minutes in the afternoon when my adrenal glands give out and recharge.

Today I have the kind of sore throat that in a gentler time I'd be sure was allergies, but now I'm all, "Did I screw up in a room?"

Also I have a thing wrong with a tooth, but I can't go and breathe on my 60-plus-year-old dentist right now. Even with PPE.

The on days are hard. In a very real way, the off days are harder.

At least when I'm on I've got something to do. I'm focused. The off days are just kind amorphous blobs. Not the gray fog of dissociative depression just yet, but hazy around the edges for sure.

When I started in burn it was hard to reintegrate into society after shifts: I had to build up this armor to function at work—and then be totally good about pulling it off and putting it away in order to have a "normal" life with other people who couldn't understand what I did.

This is like that, only so much worse. Because no one wants to talk to you about burn stuff by and large, so it's easier to put away. But now everyone has an opinion, and everyone thinks they're a scientist, and everyone's freaked out. You're just simmering in it all the time.

And like, when I was a burn nurse, you'd tell people to do things and they'd do them. They could see the burn, they were all "hold up, that's a burn," and they'd get in line.

Now, because covid's transmission is so high and so many people can be asymptomatic carriers and it hasn't affected everyone yet, you've got dumbass CEOs trying to say they've "studied" a lot and know how to fix things. (Or worse yet, the president's own kids. Come the hell on.)

So not only is it hard for me to reintegrate into society, but when I'm away from the hospital I see people out there actively making society stupider, on purpose, and for what? The economy?

Dead people don't buy much, son.

So I guess this is what I spent my cogent 30 mins of time on today. Now to stave off the existential dread until my next window sometime tomorrow afternoon.

American Association for the Advancement of Science (the

people who put out Science magazine) run an article saying that without vaccines, covid may continue through 2022. (4/14/20)

4/14/20

Man, guys. I am neither mentally nor emotionally prepared to be taking care of covid patients for the next two years.

Don't get me wrong, I 100% believe this study, which postulates covid life without vaccines. At the same time though, it makes my soul want to cry.

Like I am having a hard enough time reintegrating into society after my shifts. I need one day off and oftentimes Ativan to even begin to feel human again.

Taking care of covid patients for two more years is going to come close to breaking me.

Maybe it will; time will tell.

And it's going to break a lot of other people too, or already has. Last time I was at work, my elderly covid patient was whispering around her tube that she wanted to die. All I could give her was more propofol to zone her.

Two years of that, times every shift I have, multiplied by the people on here [Twitter] who are anti-vaxers and exponentially adjusted for the Mayor in Jaws "reopen everything!" types.

Fuck, man.

Just fuck.

I, with my relatively light patient load in California, am already burnt out. I don't know how people can expect us to keep give-give-giving for another two years of "am I geared up safely?" terror every goddamned shift.

Because it is terrifying.

It feels like you're playing Russian roulette with your life every time you take an assignment. And yeah, you do your job, because you can and no one else will. But it takes a psychic toll.

It wears on you. It's never, ever easy.

It's like trying to get 100% on a video game that has no ending and where your life actually depends on it—and the lives of your loved ones, depending on how you're isolating. And also, shit, people like my coworkers: Are they supposed to not to touch/see their kids for two years?

Fuck.

Maybe I'll talk to management and see if we can't figure out a way to go a month on/month off in the covid wing, so that month off people could at least get two weeks with their kids after their first 14 days are up.

But like, no one who has done this is going to be normal afterwards.

I got good about compartmentalizing things in the burn unit. I am a mofo when it comes to packing away Things That Should Not Be Seen. But this is far less wholesome, with far fewer saves.

I used to joke on burn that sometimes we needed a "win," and compare us to those people-scenting dogs they bring out during natural disasters.

The people that handle those dogs sometimes hide so that the dogs can find them instead of just another dead body—so that the dogs can "win," because otherwise the dogs get too sad.

In this case, we not only need to win for our patients... but we need to win for ourselves.

To know that we're personally going get out of this mess okay.

And no one can really promise that to us, without lying, until it's through.

Which makes all this pretty dang hard.

Studies show that viewing Sean Hannity's coronavirus misinformation leads to a greater number of covid-19 cases and death. (4/22/20)

Trump suggests "injecting" disinfectants as a virus cure. (4/24/20)

4/24/20

HEY YOU GUYS. Before I write fiction responsibly, but whilst the "who will drink bleach?" takes are hot, let me tell you the story of a patient who drank hand sanitizer. It is a journey.

Come with me.

So, first off, I realize my patient was drinking hand sanitizer because they were profoundly alcoholic, and not because the president had casually mentioned it to reporters on a public stage which he knew would be televised. Vast differences, yo.

But when you get your patients in, you don't always know everything. This guy was an overflow from another floor onto my burn unit; his heart was doing weird stuff and the telemetry unit was full.

He was homeless and had no belongings with him except for an extra-large Taco Bell cup. You know how Taco Bell cups are opaque white? Yeah, that.

About halfway into my night shift, this guy starts to freak out. Ripping things off of himself, wants to pace his room like a cage. I call the med resident in charge of him, because I am not a jailer, right? I'm not going to physically block someone from leaving if they want to.

Back in the olden days I was that kind of nurse, but by then I'd wisened up, because the only person who was going to get hurt in that "keep them in bed for their own good or else!" scenario was me. I did try to stop them, tried to help, gave medications, and I wheedled.

You wheel and deal a lot as a nurse. When people treat you like a waitress with access to narcotics, you get used to customer servicing. So he finally said he had to leave but that he'd be back.

I knew that wasn't true, but it gave me a chance to unplug him so he wouldn't trail IVs and wires all over the hospital. I set him free and called security. He stalks out, very deliberately taking his Taco Bell cup with him.

Talking to security, they're all 'Oh, that guy!' like they go way back, because they do, which is an inherently a bad sign. Meanwhile, I'm sitting on my unit, imagining my license fluttering off into the breeze.

Not long before that, you see, UCSF had "lost" a patient for a month.... Turns out they were dead in a stairwell, after having been presumed to have left against medical advice. So I'm all nervously awaiting a callback from security, when I get a call from another floor.

They're all, "Hey, is this guy yours?" after checking out his wristband. And I'm all, "Thank the baby Jesus, yes, keep him there," and call security to come with me to get him. The patient's much calm now—and he's still got that cup.

I forgot to mention it had a lid.

So we round him up and go back to my floor and tuck him back in, and I'm sitting there waiting. The man took the cup for something. And he's still got it now. And where I worked had a McDonald's nearby that we called the Rock Ronalds because we knew it was used for drug deals....

If he hadn't had a heart condition, I probably wouldn't have cared. Lord knows I ignored enough weed before it became legal, as long as no one tried to smoke it near oxygen. But, with the heart condition, I had to look in that cup.

So I take it from him, pop the lid off, and voila—there is an extra-large Taco Bell cup's worth of hand sanitizer inside. I realize he had to go on walkabout to find the gel pumps—our unit used the foam dispensers, which evaporated far too quickly.

I ask him, "What is this?" and he says, I shit you not: "Coconut water and protein powder," as the scent of alcohol is definitely wafting up my nose. I also forgot to mention that he's bigger than me. And that security has moved along.

I don't want to fight this dude. He'd win. And it is clear that he would fight me. So I set it down and walk out to call security again, and the resident, who finally starts "helping" by shouting at me to call poison control.

I hang out, waiting for security, watching him. He turns toward the glass wall, not even trying to hide it one whit, and decants gel hand sanitizer into his dinner meal's plastic mug and then starts adding SPLENDA.

I am watching him make a hand sanitizer daiquiri. And even though I'm scared of him, I cannot just watch him drink that. So I run in the room, grab everything, and run back outside so at least he can't corner me. And then security comes, at long last.

And "I'm a bitch!" and "that was his!" and "eff you" and "eff that." He winds up actually leaving against medical advice. I had to go back in to take his IV out while he was fuming at me, while security watched, and it was genuinely one of the scariest parts of my nursing career.

(You can't send someone out with a functional IV onto the streets. More than once we've had patients skip out on us when they realized we were going to take out their IVs, they were so happy to have access to a good vein.)

Anyhow. Poison control did answer eventually, and the

resident did come down, and yeah. I have a lot of sympathy for that guy, I do—there are alkies in my family, I get what it's like.

Just don't drink hand sanitizer—or bleach—not even if the president tells you too. BUT IF YOU MUST... use Splenda.

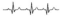

4/26/20

Just talked to my bio dad in Missouri. He's as liberal as I am & a self-aware alcoholic who works at a liquor store.

Told me today his new favorite drink was vodka with a Lysol chaser & that his store has given him a $2/hr "hazard pay" raise. I'm glad he's doing ok, for him.

4/30/20

We are down to just two positive patients in my ICU now.

I know shit is still rough in San Jose, but God bless San Francisco and Governor Newsom.

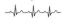

MAY 2020

One of my best friend's employers wanted their employees to just "take an antibody test" purchased from their local gym, and then come on into work if they were "safe." She asked me about that, and I thought I'd share here, too.

Here's the thing with anti-body testing so far... it's pretty dang useless for the general public to indulge in. [CA: note, this was at the time, and these were the kind of tests being distributed by gyms, etc, not done with medical supervision.]

Right now, the field seems highly unreliable, and the FDA agrees. It seems like in ten days they'll hopefully shut a lot of those test marketers down.

And even if you get a test, it'll only show you a snapshot of what's happened in your body up until that day.

I think a lot about the first patient I had at work who was in isolation for suspected covid. They wound up testing negative, hooray! And then I realized, standing there in that room with them, me still all wrapped up like a dick on prom night, that them knowing they were negative would last approximately until they left the hospital and interacted with a single other human being.

And that after that... they wouldn't really be sure anymore.

What if, though, unethical people were trying to monetize antibody tests—like they are? And making wild promises? And then those people who thought that they might have already had it started making life choices based off of that inaccurate information?

And even if you have had it—antibodies don't appear just over night. If they did, we wouldn't be getting sick, right? So there's a lag time for antibody creation that those tests won't reflect, which is another reason why getting tested is bunk.

And even if a good test showed you that you had had it... well... so what?

Do you really want to be the asshat wandering around right now without a mask, being a bad example for everyone else you pass, crowing that you're in the clear?

When we're *this* early in the science game?

When there's more than one strain of covid being actively tracked?

When you can still have particles sneezed on you by other people, who you've just encouraged to be maskless, and take them home to touch your own, possibly-with-no-anti-bodies family and friends?

You feel that confident in your decontamination procedure? 'Cause I decontaminate myself like it is *literally* my job, and I sure don't.

I understand the urge. I, too, would like some scientist to come up and rub a little lamb's blood on my forehead and say, "This plague will pass you by."

But the only actual reason the public at large needs to have antibody testing right now is so that scientists can look at data sets and prevalence studies and DO SCIENCE.

It shouldn't change how you act, and you sure as shit shouldn't be spending your hard-earned money on it. You might as well shake a magic 8 ball for all the good it'll do you.

-------〜〜〜〜-------

Trump says the people of the country should think of themselves as warriors. (5/5/20)

-------〜〜〜〜-------

5/6/2020—password-protected journal

I was driving in this morning and I saw they'd reopened the Starbucks on my way to the hospital and y'all—I miss that Starbucks. And it misses me. And I was all, well, maybe, just maybe, tomorrow....

But then my ICU just went from three covid patients to seven again today—four admits in under four hours. Two of them are in their 30s. It's still out there and it's still bad and I knew that, dammit, but like, I really was hoping, you know? Sigh.

And—I had one patient with both covid AND active TB. What the eff, man. And of course they're horribly ill and of course they're unlikely to make it, and also of course their family's unlikely to change their code status—because the family knows a family member gave it to them. Like, no one's going to want to kill a grandparent when you're the person they caught it from, you know? Talk about guilt, sheesh.

Oh, and also, I had to teach a new-grad hire today. Their first effing day. Talk about jumping—or being pushed into—the deep end.

5/7/20

Work is so worky today, y'all.

We're short, we're proning three pts, and have paralyzed a fourth.

I like teaching (my new hire is back today), but everything is shortcut city because of how behind we are just trying to get shit done, and I feel like that's not going well.

Bleh.

5/7/20—later in the day

It's bad enough worrying I'm bringing covid home to my husband, but I'm watching this brand-new nurse who didn't even get to practice isolating on MRSA and C. diff patients before working covid patients with me.

I love to teach and that's why they picked me, but I should've refused yesterday, in hindsight.

[CA: MRSA and C. diff are other illnesses that patients are frequently in isolation for. They're dangerous, but not often deadly.]

I've actually thought about this moment a lot since it happened, since in hindsight I feel it was one of the most unethical things I've ever done.

My hospital decided to train up a few fresh nursing school grads, just in case we got overwhelmed and needed the extra nurses on hand.

I'm not entirely sure what the thought process was behind that—I guess we couldn't siphon off other nurses internally from the hospital to train up, since they were needed on their own floors?

But there's no way to crash-course a new grad into being an ICU nurse, really.

And there's no way I should've accepted him following me into a covid room that day.

It's one thing for me to risk my life for a job that I signed up for, that I've got fourteen years of experience doing.

But to bring a new grad, who'd never gowned up like their life depended on it before, into the abattoir with me?

That was a shit thing to do, and I've regretted it ever since.

We kept him and a few like him around for a few weeks, and then I guess we released them back into the wild.

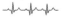

Trump's valet has coronavirus, as does one of Pence's staffers. (5/7/20)

5/8/20

Trying not to be a bitch here so my husband won't make me delete this again, but I hope THE RIGHT LESSONS ARE LEARNED.

Yesterday, we enrolled my covid patient in a case study for a new medication, and a relative of their family member (who also has covid and who gave it to them)—called me to beg me to put them in the trial too.

They weren't doing well and they were scared and—that shouldn't be happening.

People should not be calling asking to be put on experimental drugs. Least of all calling me for that.

And then they were all, "Hey, I just want to let you know, if I die, here's the next person who gets to make choices for 'patient'."

They sounded like shit on the phone.

I couldn't offer medical advice.

I just listened to them cry as they tried to figure out who was going take care of their relative's medical decisions if they themselves died, and told them to please go into get help if they needed it.

This whole situation is bogus and bullshit, so if it takes key members of the GOP getting sick or exposed to see substantive useful action, then go-virus-go.

And if they're unwilling to act after this, well then... I hope the virus works a little bit harder to clear the path to sanity.

(As an aside, my husband doesn't "make" me do anything—he just knows I have a temper and frequently counsels against me making an ass of myself in public & I've learned to listen to him. Unless I'm still pissed off 24 hrs. later, heh.)

[CA: my husband is a much nicer person than I am, and occasionally his goodness rubs off on me.]

5/10/2020—password protected journal

Took care of a mom in her 40's today. Nothing else going on going on for her, healthwise, just covid.

I'd be hella surprised if she lives. She's already on two pressors to keep her blood pressure up, 90% oxygen, and we have her breathing at 36 times a min, which is a lot. Her PEEP is already 12, and the normal for that is five. So yeah.

All this talk of opening again—and seeing all those people out at Mother's Day brunches—goddamn.

5/10/20

Look Twitter-friends: maybe, assuming you still have disposable income, which I know is tight, you could buy my book.

I'd like to go down to only having one job that terrifies me, and publishing is safer.

I'm in the breakroom at work trying not to have a panic attack.

[CA: I write paranormal romances as Cassie Alexander and under a shared penname. There'll be links at the back of this book for the curious.]

5/10/20

Hey, so, you should finalize all the legal shit you can now, so that the spouse you're married to in name alone isn't making your medical decisions/dodging our calls.

If you don't want them in your life, you probably don't want them in charge of your health.

[CA: more than once during covid we had family members actively dodge our palliative care team's Goals of Care calls, because they didn't want to talk about the possibility of their loved one dying.]

5/10/20

My patient has precisely one parameter left on their ventilator that I can go up on.

Everything else is maxed.

They are younger than I am.

No comorbidities.

5/10/20

I'm really tired of this new normal.

I don't want to get used to it.

I can't survive if I don't, though.

Have I survived?

This is as good a time as any to ask that of myself.

Is this survival?

I walk, I talk, I breathe.

But somedays I'm just a fine mist that everything else feels like it can pass through.

Other times I'm so solid and the weight of being me is so much, I can't even get out of bed. I feel like I could sink into the center of the earth.

I know that I should take advantage of the opportunities that I've been given.

After all, I'm still alive.

Right?

The White House has directed all West Wing staff to wear masks at all times in the building, except when they are at their own desks. (5/11/20)

5/12/20

Been seeing a lot of "if masks work, why do businesses need to be closed—and if they don't work, why are we forced to wear them?" posts on FB lately. Here's an analogy you can use to shut that line of logic down.

So, real talk—masks aren't 100% perfect. But they're about risk mitigation.

It's the difference between having sex while tracking ovulation vs. using condoms vs. using birth control.

Using the logic of the example given above, just because sometimes people get pregnant on birth control (99.7% effective!), no one should use birth control.

But you and I both know that that's not right. No one using birth control would go off of it because of a 0.03% risk it won't work. No one using birth control wants to get pregnant.

And—no one wants to die of covid.

I know it's frustrating, especially when there's no universal basic income, which I absolutely believe the government should be doing as a trade-off for all of us essentially "practicing abstinence," AKA staying at home, which is effing hard, and we all know how well it works long term....

But masks work.

And staying home works even better!

So, failing our ability to stay home, if science says I should keep my mask on to try to save people's lives... that's an easy choice. Easy peasy, done.

⎯⎫⎪⎫⎪⎫⎯

5/13/20

Can't tell if I'm burnt out at work or have work-related PTSD, the Cassie Alexander life story.

Trump says that nurses are "running into death like soldiers run into bullets." (5/14/20)

5/14/20

I regret to tell y'all, but I'm genuinely uninterested in dying for most of my patients.

Have I done stupid shit and run into dangerous rooms before? Yeah.

Do I want to have to, though? Oh hell no.

Also... running into death is never beautiful.

Who the hell watches a WWII film and cheers FOR THE FUCKING BULLETS?

Talk about our grace or empathy or resilience under the shittiest conditions most of us have ever known.

But don't say our possibly dying is beautiful.

What the absolute fuck.

5/15/2020—personal journal

My parents visited today for our anniversary, so we did a socially-distanced-and-with-masks hang out in my backyard.

We brushed up so close to political stuff—my mom thinks this'll all be over in a few months and they're planning on going to Texas in October so my dad can walk a friend's daughter who they're close to down the aisle. According to my dad, we "can't hold back the world forever."

Sigh.

I tried to explain things to them, but they at least say they're good about wearing masks and I do believe them on that front.

The rest of the lessons'll come soon enough. I hope they bought refundable tickets.

5/17/20—password protected journal

My mom messaged me today to tell me that I seemed depressed. I was all, YOU THINK?

And also, yo, mom, it's called PTSD.

Because every time I go into work I want to cry or throw up, and it's all endless all the time because people can't keep their damn masks on because of "freedoms!"

Like I could handle any time-delineated thing—if it was all, yo, Cassie, handle this shit for three years—aye, aye, cap'n—I totally could. But I don't think I can deal with the not knowing.

I tried to share this with my mom, only calmer, and she doesn't get it. Or get the cognitive dissonance I experience. She used to be a teacher, so I wish I'd thought of this metaphor sooner—it'd be if she were expected to teach in a classroom just down the hall from an active shooter. Just carry on like normal. While people were out there getting shot, and you could hear the shots, but other people were pretending it wasn't happening and you weren't allowed to leave. Oh, and, by the way, now they're trying to also erase our coworkers' retirement funds.

But just keep working, just keep working!

So I spent the past three hours in a panic attack because a) work, tomorrow and b) not feeling seen. Again. I don't know why I ever expect any differently. It feels like my parents couldn't pick me out of a lineup.

I know I disappoint them. I'm their overly intelligent spiky child. The one who's too hard to hold because she's busy telling you all the ways that you're wrong. They don't want to hear that they're wrong, and I don't blame them; I can't imagine that it's fun for them. But at the same time, I don't want to pretend that they're right, ever again. Especially when the things they want to be right on, Trump, masks, etc., are things that are actively putting me in danger, over and over.

The thought of pretending to be nice—science? What science?—makes me want to hurl. So I'm not entirely sure where that leaves them and me, again.

Anyhow.

Sometimes it's good for me to go to work and get away from things. But this isn't one of those times—I wouldn't want me as a nurse tomorrow. My head is Not in The Game. So I called in sick.

I just hope I figure out a way to not waste tomorrow—I'm not sure what I'll be doing, but hopefully something good, even if it's just gardening again.

Going to go take another Ativan. Sleep a real sleep. Hopefully wake up in a better mood, or more focused, or less terrified.

5/24/20

Five out of the eight patients in the ED right now are in covid isolation. If I don't put a fresh battery in my work phone here and it runs out, I can't admit, right?

5/25/20

Well WTF guys!!! My intubated covid patient from Mother's Day got successfully extubated!!!!

JUNE 2020

6/2/20—excerpt from my author newsletter

Hey so... I always wonder how political to get in these newsletters. As you can imagine, I have pretty strident feelings about public health, and public health being politicized was absolutely nowhere on my "things that'll happen in 2020" bingo card, but here we are.

So, um, go buy one of my books before you possibly get cranky at me, BUT HERE GOES.

Back when I was on the burn unit, we had this conundrum with patient's families, especially when a patient's injuries were "incompatible with life." Families always wanted to see their loved ones, totally understandably, you know? No one wants to believe that you're going to lose someone; it is too awful to comprehend—especially when the person is still *right there!*

So we'd have people who were 80% burned, definitely not going to survive, but we'd do full dressings on them, making them look like the Michelin man with gauze, so that the families could see them one last time and be there with them when they passed.

The problem with that was when people didn't get it—I mean, they were looking at their loved one, and sure, they were really wrapped up in gauze, but they could see their face or maybe hold a hand, so how could they really be dying?

The easiest way to get conditions across would've been to show the loved one the dying person's injuries. To lift the dressings up. But —that would've irreparably scarred the family member. They would understand, but in pursuit of their understanding, our actions would be untheraupetic—even cruel. They'd probably have PTSD or intrusive thoughts about the horrors that they saw for the rest of their life. Even when you work there, you can't erase seeing those types of things, you can only contextualize them. Because you are helping people the vast majority of the time, it keeps the nightmares at bay. Mostly.

So we'd tell the family members no, and keep watch—because people would try to peek—and let them be there at the end, while telling them that there was nothing we could possibly do about it, we were sorry, truly.

And I think about that a lot now, in our "I've got to see it with my own two eyes!" society that we're in. About how people can't believe what they see unless it happens, and profoundly enough at that, to someone they know. How sometimes people don't want to wear masks until they're personally affected by covid, and oftentimes by then it's too late—they've already exposed so many others.

I spend a lot of time wondering how to counteract that. Mandatory corpse viewings? Grabbing someone by the back of the neck and making them look through an ICU window? How can we prove something as awful as covid to someone who won't believe it unless they are personally traumatized by it?

[CA: I and many of my other coworkers said during this time period that if any of us got covid, we wanted our care to be fully streamed. I would've been A-OK with the entire internet watching me get my ass wiped if it meant someone else realizing that covid was a real, real thing.]

I was at work on Mother's Day, taking care of a mother who was younger than I was, with two blood pressure medications running, her vent settings maxed, so much that we were worried we might pop a lung, and she was proned to maximize her access to her good lung tissue. And then on break I was looking at my phone at that brunch place in Denver that was open for the holiday, gleefully flouting the local laws, people packed in.

I wanted to throw up. My cognitive dissonance and moral distress were off the charts. (This is why I write sexy dragon-shifter books in my free time. I want to live in a sexy dragon-shifter world where things make sense and plots happen for reasons.)

Anyhow—I don't have an answer for that. It's just that the situations feel similar to me now. And it's frustrating, because I guarantee you these people don't want to see what I see. But they seem incapable of imagining it—or trusting me and others like me that it happens.

I know wearing masks, especially as summer heats up, is going suck. I totally get you. But there's a reason that countries that've worn them have shown consistent declines in covid cases. Masks really do work. And as science moves on and we feel more confident that surface contact transmission is low—it's all 'bout them droplets, baybee—masks are HUGELY effective in stopping those.

If you see anyone freaking out about CO_2 retention, well, that's bogus. I wear a mask all day long at work—as do hundreds of thousands of people in multiple occupations, even prior to this—and it's fine. I do have a lot of sympathy for people who masks freak out—I think that one woman we all saw crying on Twitter about wearing a mask was having a panic attack, for sure.

But like, I'm taking Ativan on my off days now to control my own panic disorder, which this situation is making ding off the charts. If that's you, get treatment, for sure; anxiety disorders are no joke. But having one isn't an excuse to risk other people's lives.

You wouldn't go to a buffet without a sneezeguard, would you? Heck no.

So why would you face the outside world without one right now, when there's stuff out there a lot worse than boogers in the potato salad?

Okay, that's enough. I lecture because I love. I don't want to see any more people at work with this than I have to.

I'll lay off the soapbox for a few newsletters and go back to sexy manbeasts, swear!

<3
Cassie

—‍⎯‍⌁‍⎯‍

6/11/2020—personal journal

The only thing that's going to dig us out of this (prior to a vaccine being available) is 100% mandatory mask wearing.

Unfortunately, there's just not enough political willpower to do so.

I mean they were chasing down the public health official in Orange County—they doxxed her and she retired early because of assholes....

It's going to get a lot a lot worse before it gets better.

[CA: "doxing" is when you put someone's personal information on the internet so that they can be harassed.]

6/14/20

Somedays I just really want someone to tell me that's it's going to be okay.

But I also don't want anyone to lie to me.

6/14/20—excerpt from author newsletter

Does it feel like everywhere is reopening now? Or is that just me? I know California is slowly loosening things up.

I have a friend who works at a hair salon. The salon itself went and put all this plexiglass in to protect people and limited their seating, etc., doing everything it could do to get ready to reopen.

But one of the ladies there didn't want to wear a mask to work—and went as far out as to get a doctor's note that said she couldn't wear a mask and then tried to sue the salon to make accommodations, under the ADA.

Fraudulent lawsuits aside—and that women wound up just getting let go—it made me think about things even more than I already do (which is A LOT) and come up with a list of possible medical reasons that people might be able to get a doctor's note to not wear a mask with, and they're mostly respiratory issues: asthma, COPD.

But here's the kicker with those:

If you have asthma or COPD and you get covid because you didn't want to wear a mask?

You're pretty much signing on for long-term ventilator time.

Covid isn't any nicer to your lungs because you had an excuse to be maskless, honestly. And I remember a few weeks ago there were people who'd printed things off the internet, claiming that there were also medical exceptions and that no one could ask them because of HIPAA (aka the Health Information Privacy Act).

That's not how that works—HIPAA only covers health, and health-adjacent organizations, that're dealing with medical information.

Not your grocery store.

I mean by that same token, if you were going play that card, someone who was bleeding from a knife wound could wander around an entire grocery store, spilling blood everywhere and shouting "HIPAA!" any time anyone asked him to leave. Or, to be more gross but to hammer the point home—someone could be uncontrollably shitting due to a medical condition, but you can't just shout "HIPAA!" and expect that to get you out of trouble when you've got diarrhea in the frozen food aisle, you know?

Anyhow, everyone I've talked to with pre-existing lung issues among my friends group (people with asthma, CF, etc.), they're all scared to leave the house and/or would never not wear a mask, because they know far, far better than most how important their lungs are. So I give anyone who says they "can't wear a mask" a huge side-eye.

Now—back to the WHO! [CA: the World Health Organization, an international coalition dedicated to attaining "the highest possible level of health" for all people.]

I know the WHO confused a lot of people by putting out data earlier in the week that said asymptomatic people rarely transmit covid—which is true(ish...see studies referenced below)!

BUT—just because you're asymptomatic currently doesn't mean you're not presymptomatic.

Asymptomatic people are people who have covid and who literally never have any symptoms from it.

Presymptomatic people are people who have covid who CURRENTLY don't have any symptoms from it. But you can still transmit covid!

How can you tell if you're asymptomatic vs presymptomatic?

YOU CAN'T. Not really.

Because to know if you currently have covid you'd need to be tested (which you likely wouldn't think of doing if you had no symptoms) and/or you'd need to wait 3-14 days to see if symptoms kick up.

So yes, the WHO statement was technically true for their current small data sets, but it was also wildly unhelpful in the current climate, especially given the rate of medical illiteracy in the US right now.

There's an article coming out from the CDC in Sept that states that most of the clusters in Japan came from young people, from 20-

39, who had no symptoms, and a lot of those transmissions occurred the day before the person felt they had symptoms—so they thought they were asymptomatic, but in reality they were just presymptomatic.

So please don't stop wearing masks because you don't "feel bad" or whatever. You could still be killing someone. Really, I mean it.

I know it's SO TEMPTING to feel like our government is run by sane people who have our best interests at heart, but that's not the case currently, alas. Right now I feel like a lot of us are in an abusive relationship with the government, in so many more ways than just this one, where we want to believe in them because why would they want more people than have ever died in any war so far to die?

That's where we're going. Them's the stats.

Do you realize if they get more than 50 cases in South Korea, they shut everything back down? They treat every life there like a treasure. And it really chaps my hide—no, that's too light, more like it breaks my soul—that we don't seem to have that same wherewithal here.

I saw someone on Twitter recently refer to the Stock Market as the "Rich People's Feelings Graph" and, yeah. To a lot of rich people, the money they make is worth more than your shot at life. And not even just life-life, but like a satisfying and whole one. Because surviving covid doesn't mean you're not left with lung damage, etc., to deal with for forever, you know?

Take a second and follow this link for me—[CA: link to covidexit-strategy.org removed]. It's graphs and data from daily covid trends, drawn directly from the CDC.

What you'll notice about the first picture, even if that's the only one you hit—is that NO WAY NO HOW should most states be reopening. According to guidelines from the White House, you'd need two weeks of declining cases for reopening to be appropriate. If you scroll down that site again… how many states look like they're currently on a decline? Not that many, alas.

But the Rich People's Feelings Graph needs to be fed, so here we are.

Here comes that positive note I promised above though!

Remember that hair salon, where two hairdressers saw 146 people and then found out later they had active, symptomatic, covid?

Well, out of the 41 people they saw who opted to get tested too—not a one of them had covid!

Why?

BECAUSE THEY HAD MASKS ON!!!! MASKS WORKKKKKKKK!!!!

And remember—a mask that doesn't cover your nose is just a chin hammock! That ain't masking!

<3

Cassie

⎯⎯ᜎᜎ⎯⎯

I'M INTERRUPTING from the present day to explain to you the title of this book, seeing as I just mentioned the WHO, the World Health Organization, which Trump pulled us out of, and Biden put us back into.

Each year they designate it to be a "year of the something," and 2020 was—I'm not shitting you—the Year of the Nurse. I think it was the 200th anniversary of Nightingale's birthday or something.

So each and every one of us across America had posters in our hospitals, somewhere in a breakroom, announcing 2020: YEAR OF THE NURSE as the walls started caving in.

In fact, 2020 was so bad we got a redo. 2021 is also, officially, the YEAR OF THE NURSE.

I figured it sounded plenty dramatic for a title, especially for a somewhat chronological journal like this one—but also that any healthcare worker drifting by who survived last year would see it and be in on the "joke," given how 2020 went and how 2021 is so far going.

California institutes its mask mandate. (6/18/20)

6/21/20

My mom doesn't understand why I can't visit.
   sigh
When am I going to be able to really hang out with my folks again?

6/22/20

It is quite a thing to never look forward to going to your job again.

6/22/20—later in the day

I lied earlier.
   I still like my job (some shifts!)
   I just really hate mornings.
   (Although I'm getting beaten like a rented mule here today and my hand is bruised from pushing bicarb.)

6/24/20

Everyone had masks on at the Home Depot today. It was a glorious thing.
   For the first time in a long time, I actually felt hopeful.
   Yes, I broke my bubble to go to HD. I garden for mental health reasons, so I had to pick my poison.
   [CA: I made sure to wear n95s when out amongst the public, and this trip to Home Depot was my first non-

work/pharmacy/grocery store/gas station trip since 3/11. I took isolating very seriously, as befit someone coming into contact with covid patients.]

6/26/20

The only thing I'm actually looking forward to that's covid-19 related is when we get to the stage that Italy did when the mayors go on the news and threaten people with flamethrowers etc. for going outside.

I give it... two weeks.

Three, on the outside.

[CA: this was an actual, beautiful, thing that happened in Italy at the coronavirus's peak there. Italian mayors ran around threatening to use weapons, chastising citizens for being outdoors after curfew. There's a link to more information in the ancillary materials.]

6/28/2020—personal journal

I am laser-angry again. My patient this past weekend was an almost 80-yr-old grandparent. Their family had a Memorial Day party and one of their guests was feeling sick. They went and got a covid test and then, instead of waiting for the results, they went to the party anyways. Turns out they did indeed have covid and gave it to my patient.

So now, this person—who was in all other respects very healthy, might die, or at least have their end-of-life quality significantly diminished, and if it goes in a comfort-care direction their family's never going to want to pull the plug because whoever gave him covid is going to feel guilty for straight up killing him.

Because they did.

It's so messed up.

6/28/20

I just had a Trump supporting respiratory therapist tell me anti-mask stuff while wearing an n95 and call me "emotional" for calling them out on it.

We're all going to die... starting with this dude because I may kill him.

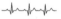

6/30/20—personal journal

The bleak is very vast today and uncomfortably tenacious.

I'm cracking a little.

I'm very tired of having to be so strong all the time. I'm looking at the news reports and this shit is going to be never-ending. I'm already burnt and it's not going to get better anytime soon. There's no light at the end of the tunnel, nothing real or solid to look forward to.

Even though my hospital isn't overwhelmed yet, they're already bringing sick people from Los Angeles up to Stanford, so if we've got capacity and southern California shits the bed, we're next in line.

None of this had to happen. No one wanted to listen. One day I'm a "hero" (which I don't want to be), the next on Twitter I'm getting called a slut for telling people to wear masks.

It's exhausting giving a shit. I'm good at my job, and my administration would still gladly dick me over if they could. My parents still think going on a trip in August—with my aunt and uncle who live in Arizona—is a great idea. No one wants to listen or cares if other people survive, or if I have be the tragic iPad facetime jockey so people can pretend to have a moment with someone who is intubated and sedated and non-reactive to them.

I love the world. It's why I do this.

I hate the world for what it's doing to me.

I'm not sure who I'm going to be at the end of all this. I hope I like her. I hope she's still me. But I don't think I can get through without caring less, just to protect myself, and man that feels shitty.

How do I mete out enough compassion to properly function as a nurse, but not so much that I lose myself, become more broken, or turn into a bitter shell?

I don't know how to work that dial. I can usually bounce back with a day off and gardening. But my bounce is getting stiffer and the boxes I compartmentalize all my shit into are getting very full.

Hopefully another benzo tonight does the trick.

Goldman-Sachs estimates a national mask mandate could've saved one trillion dollars. (6/30/20)

JULY 2020

7/1/20

We're not even done clearing out our patients from Memorial Day gatherings and here comes 4th of July.

7/1/20

Long, long day with my first patient (covid plus a trip to CT) and here comes my admit....

But that's okay.

I can keep anyone alive for 2.5 hrs. unless God's personally calling them home.

cracks knuckles

7/1/2020—password protected journal

My hospital's on the list to receive overflow covid-positive prisoners from San Quentin.

I actually don't mind prisoners as patients, but this just goes to show how we're all interconnected, and how my coworkers and I are trapped.

Bad decisions elsewhere will float up and get us eventually.

Nowhere's safe.

7/2/20—password protected journal

I am not doing well. Woke up to kick the cats out right now and segued straight into a panic attack.

I'm trying to keep it together (or at least quiet, heh) till my husband gets up at eight.

I hate being a mess in assorted places on the internet, but oh well. My real-life [CA: my girls' chat] friend group doesn't have much bandwidth right now because one of my best friends' mothers is dying and she needs us more. I cried on the phone with D last night and almost barfed everything over E in chat, but it was almost midnight and I didn't want people's phones to ring with my nonsense.

I just need some love, y'all. This is so awful and it's not going anywhere. I feel so trapped and forgotten. I almost had a panic attack at work yesterday—luckily, heh, my patient crumped right afterwards and I laser-focused on them.

So now I'm sitting here, sobbing silently, typing this on my phone.

I don't have a good way to end it, either.

7/2/20—password protected journal, later the same day

General trigger warning for suicide talk, sorry.

My husband brought me avocado toast (because we're Californian, heh). I slept in, plus or minus assorted cat shenanigans, till 11, and then he made me eat again, and gave me no shit about announcing that I'm going to Home Depot to get dirt today.

I've been here before. I know how to do the things. Reach out for help (to the right people. Not my family). Take the meds, eat, drink, exercise, sunlight, etc.

My husband's and my inside joke regarding suicide is that he knows I'm suicidal if I want to write poetry.

I read this book by a neuroscientist who had had a traumatic experience and became hypergraphic afterwards—then she studied the relationships between creativity and the brain, and apparently poets are way more at risk for that sort of thing. (Again, this is according to this book I read once ten years ago, so who the hell knows. But it explains vast tracts of time in my teens, heh.)

The downer of actually knowing that about myself is that I don't actually get to write any poetry because that's usually my Red Alert, and I try to pull up rather than hanging out in that bad-for-me headspace.

The flip side is that, prior to learning that about myself, I've got dated, poignant reminders of every time I've ever been really badly off before.

So here's the last poem I wrote back in 2014, when I also wanted to die:

> *Oh my love don't weep for me,*
> *The time for tears is past.*
> *If you've done what I've asked you to,*
> *We'll be together soon at last.*

Don't let the willow hear you cry,
Or bruise ferns as you tread,
If you've done what I've asked you to,
Then our love isn't dead.

Don't look for me inside of tombs,
Or underneath cold stone,
Don't search for me in crumbled soil,
You'll only dig up bones.

None of death's trappings, my love
Hold meaning anymore.
When one such as I and one such as you,
Are divided by death's door.

As long as you've done what I've asked,
You know my heart is true.
Only bury me with bolt cutters,
And I'll return to you.

YESTERDAY'S POEM was going to be called What to Do When the Light Ends, but that's as far as I got.

[CA: the book is *The Midnight Disease: The Drive to Write, Writer's Block, and the Creative Brain,* by Alice W. Flaherty]

7/5/20

Look, all I really want in this world is for you all to survive all this and for you not to endanger me, my family, friends, and coworkers.

Just by wearing a simple piece of fabric.
I don't get why that's so hard.

7/9/20

I don't know how to explain to people that they should give a shit.

7/10/20

My personal, equally valid and equally calming self-care choices today are to shop for plants or read Wikipedia pages about serial killers.

7/10/2020—personal journal

My 70-plus-comorbidities-out-the-wazoo aunt and uncle who live in Arizona are still going to visit my 70-plus parents (same same) and they're all going to go to a casino in Tahoe together to hang out at the end of the month.

Lolsob

Also had the world's most depressing conversation with my mother last night, re: kids essentially being disposable, and school reopenings (because why not open schools after there were protests?)

I really hate this post-truth society thing we're living in.

[CA: Black Lives Matter protests did not increase local covid stats because they were outdoors and, by and large, protestors properly wore masks. See ancillary material for more information.]

7/12/2020—personal journal

My husband, who has dutifully not left the house since March 10th, finally went to go see his mother at her memory care facility yesterday. They only recently started allowing visitation with strict rules.

Of course people with Alzheimer's aren't good about keeping masks on, and his mom had a cough... and today that facility is closing down because one of the residents there has covid.

I'm really glad I gave him one of my spare n95's and fit it to him the night before, and he wears glasses and... yeah.

He's all upset about his mom right now, whereas I'm all worried about him, heh.

7/11/20

It's rich when people who have 20 years more to live, max, are so invested in selling out kids who could have 80.

7/12/20

If your economy requires a river of human blood to survive, consider instead that it's already broken.

7/13/20—excerpt from author newsletter

Hey, so—first off, I hope ALLLLLLLLL of you all are well and that every single dang person you know is well, too.

This is going to be a rather long email, and I apologize for that— but people keep saying they like the science and opinions! Just be warned (for people who've recently joined up), there will be a time when I go back to talking about paranormal romance and hot dragon-shifters again!

I'm sorry I fell off the face of the earth there for a bit. I was dealing with some pretty severe depression, because everything felt endless. And it seems to me (from keeping an eye on Twitter at least) that I've been about two-three weeks ahead of the national mood, so I figured now was a good time to reach out again, because I bet a lot of y'all are getting depressed too.

Why?

Mostly because it seems like this thing is never going to end.

So let's talk about that a bit.

I hope by now everyone is really convinced that masks work, and are worthwhile, and please-for-the-love-of-god need to cover your entire nose and mouth (don't make me cut you). They remain our cheapest and best defense against this thing. Please use them every time you leave your house. I don't care how good your neighbors/friends/relatives/loved ones claim they're being.

Honestly, it'll be safer for you if you just treat everyone else you know like a liar who licked every doorknob on the way to see you. I hate to say "be paranoid"—but we're in this for the long haul.

So yes, please, be paranoid.

Survive.

But let's talk about what it's going to take to beat this thing.

In addition to a mass commitment to wearing a mask literally all the time indoors and almost all of the time outdoors....

We really need to give people money to stay home. More money. Legitimate amounts of money.

I just want to put this idea into your head and then explain myself. And I know some people are sore about this (my mother among them, who thinks that people who're "unemployed" are getting too much money... no matter the fact that she's been retired since she was 55, which is a dream that literally no one of my generation can even imagine having).

But—until you give people an economic incentive to stay home and the ability to stay home, we're never going to break the virus's back—we're going to be stuck in this hellish freefall until there's a vaccine. The schools are never really going to be able to open (more on that later), and neither are colleges, and neither are the restaurants and small businesses that keep a community alive.

The people who are afraid of giving us money to ride this out and fight it successfully are THE SAME PEOPLE who say we need to get "back to work!" or we'll all "wind up depressed!" (newsflash: many of us already are) and we'll "break the economy!"

My friend, if your economy requires a hundred thousand PREVENTABLE DEATHS to survive... it's already broken. Defund the military a little or tax Bezos more or some shit—figure it out. Because what we're going to have for the next few months is in no way shape or form going to resemble the type of "economy!" we all need in order to be a functioning society.

Why?

The dying, mostly. Or the fear of dying.

We're going to end up with a generation of people really scarred by this. Because when you find out that your loved one died because someone else "had" to go to work (or "had" to go to Disney World, hang on) that's going to eff you up pretty bad. More so since you're not going to be able to visit them in the hospital when they do die.

There's two levels to all of this—

First, people need to be able to afford to stay home, and second, people should (as much as possible) be made to stay home, and nothing pretty much exemplifies that more than the fact that Disney World just opened yesterday.

I love me some Disney. I used to have annual passes, I've got an embarrassing amount of Maleficent collectibles, etc., so it pains me to talk smack about them, but....

Disney World has absolutely no business being open.

The people who are visiting there are endangering themselves needlessly (and, through that, everyone else they know and/or will come in contact with for the next two weeks) AND the people who work there... do they really want to be there right now? Would they be working there if they had any other financial choice?

Florida just broke the daily record for one-day increases in covid cases in the US.

We need to make it so that the people who work for Disney don't starve to death or end up evicted while doing the right thing and staying home.

And we need to disincentivize this kind of opportunity for spread, for as long as there are foolishly selfish people out there willing to spread it.

You see, what worked in other countries was intense contact tracing—if scientists knew where you were and who you were with, they could work backwards from there and get all of those people to quarantine. Everyone sits home for two weeks—PAID FOR TWO WEEKS. FED FOR TWO WEEKS—and voila, the virus loses its chance to transmit and disappears.

Right now, the way we're running things, we're kind of fucked.

We're still allowed to be too mobile. We're too scared of government surveillance. We lie about where we've been too much. Hell, we apparently go to "covid parties"!

Here's how stuff is going to go down:

The next two-three weeks are going to be full of people wishing they hadn't done what they did. And we're going to get a lot of news on Facebook about how people who refused to wear masks are horribly ill or the 4th of July party everyone attended killed Grandma and hospitalized four.

And then after that... school's supposed to start?

I don't think so.

Right now—we "need" school to start because we need someplace to babysit our kids (the education's just a side benefit)—so that people can work. Which is why we need to be paying people to NOT WORK. So they can stay home with their kids.

We can make up a grade later, nationally. What we can't do is replace human lives.

We can't ask teachers to put themselves on the front lines—AGAIN! Because, as I saw going around on Twitter yesterday—how the hell are teachers supposed to do active shooter drills with social distancing? Come on!

I know there are theoretical ways that we could make things "safe" enough for kids to go back into classrooms, but you and I both know the state of public education in this country, with teachers crowdfunding pencils. Let's not kid ourselves that the building down the street, built in the 70s, is going to double in size and/or get a new HVAC in time for August.

So we, as a nation, need to suck it up buttercup and GIVE PEOPLE MONEY TO SURVIVE. Two-three months would stop covid dead in its tracks, or get it down to numbers that could be testable/traceable again.

There's no reason that we can't do this now, and if we don't do it now, because of the current administration, well... brace yourselves for us to have to do it come Jan 2021 (I fervently hope and pray) but only after countless other deaths that didn't have to happen.

I was going to talk about POLSTs and end-of-life care, but this has already gotten too long, and probably too depressing. And I'm sorry I keep sending these weird public health emails that have nothing to do with paranormal romance at all. I know that's not what y'all signed-up for.

I just really want everyone to make it through this thing alive, whatever it takes.

<3
Cassie

Trump says, "Think of this: If we didn't do testing—instead of testing over 40 million people, if we did half the testing, we'd have half the cases. If we did another—you cut that in half, you'd have yet again half of that." (7/14/20)

7/14/20

PS: the mooooood at my hospital today. We've done nothing but work hard and b*tch about Trump.

7/16/20—email to members of my family, in response to my mom saying, "Everyone has opinions about covid," because I know both my brother and I were laying into her.

I'm going to ignore most of this email, but I do want to say one thing, to both of y'all, as kindly as possible, after this quote from you, mom: "Everyone has opinions about covid."

Mom, what if I told you, "Everyone has opinions about the French horn." (Bro, pretend that's "has opinions about how to fight fires" and use your imagination.)

And then that all of a sudden, people all over the world—none of them musicians, mind you—were all, "No! You blow into the bell end of the French horn! That's the only way to make it work!"

And you'd be all, "What the heck are you talking about? I've been playing the French horn for 60 years! You use the mouthpiece, dummies!"

But they would be all, "Nope! I saw it on TV! The President said to blow into the bell end. He yells at musicians who tell him to use the mouthpiece! Also, there's these videos on YouTube I've been watching, and all of them say, bell-end only, from here on out!"

You'd be sitting there a little stunned and boggled, wouldn't you be?

Because, as a professional musician, you would know you were right.

There's only one way to play the French horn. The right way. With the mouthpiece.

Well, that's how I feel every day now, reading the news about how people are treating covid, still going around outside, and not wanting to wear masks.

With all due respect to the both of you—neither of you are as professional in this as I am, or have had your eyes as intently on the ball for the past 4 months. Remember how I emailed you on 3/9, Mom? To say "news out of Italy is bad, grab groceries and stay in!" I've been watching this situation on the ground like a hawk, like it's my job, because it is.

It's my profession.

I cannot help that the president and Fox news have been lying about covid all this time. But that doesn't turn my science into "opinions." I despair of the fact that we now live in a post-truth society where anyone can make up stuff and post it online. But... science is science, truly. You can try to blow into the bell end all you want, but you're still not going to get a good tone, and you know that.

Unfortunately, sometimes science does change. That's it's nature. That's actually the whole point of science—to change and grow as we learn more. But what this means is that if you're going to participate in scientific culture, you've got to really keep your eye on the ball. So Bro, I know you were talking about herd immunity in Sweden—well, that data's a month old, and their major scientists who chose to try herd immunity out realize that they made their mortality rates far higher there than other countries. And herd immunity's a dream at this point. It would cause so many deaths, plus recent studies have shown that covid antibodies don't stay in your body long enough to prevent a second infection (just do a Google search for covid antibodies herd immunity and see). So there's no actual hope for herd immunity at this point in time. (Notice how I say "at this point in time," though—because if some real science comes out and backs that, I'd be effing thrilled.)

Any time I ever say anything that's "science based" on any of my feeds, I know I have an obligation to look things up and make sure that whatever I'm talking about is based on the freshest data from the most trusted sources, because people trust me and I have a professional obligation not to let them down.

I'm sorry I keep telling both of you news you don't want to hear. For what it's worth—I don't want to hear it either! I don't like thinking I'm going to be in the trenches dealing with this for the next year AT ALL. In fact, guess what?!?! NO ONE WANTS TO HEAR GOOD NEWS MORE THAN ME. But I also refuse to have non-scientific smoke blown up my ass.

When all this started going down, I called you, Bro, scared shitless about not having enough gear to do my job, and you told me, "Well quit!" all spitefully (a thing I don't think you've ever apologized for). Like quitting and getting to live in my house that I love and keeping the health insurance that I need as an American because our health insurance sucks was such an easy option. So thanks for all your compassion then.

And do you remember when I called you crying, Mom, because we were running out of gowns and I was scared? This was around Easter, for the 12hr shift when I had two covid patients and had been given three gowns, that I needed to share also with respiratory therapy and janitorial, no less. The shift that I had to go and find chemo gowns to use and re-use in the room for myself (such a not safe thing), so I could give the plastic ones to my other people. And I don't remember what you said, something about "Oh, it's not that bad, you'll get gear" to me—the day after one of the most traumatizing shifts I'd ever had because I'd felt scared and I'm pretty sure I hung up on you, too? (And then called my BFF and talked to her for an hour because she didn't downplay my concerns and was actually worried about me and would listen to me?)

I don't know why either of you credit people who tell you to blow into the bell-end of the French horn more than you do me.

This entire time the both of you haven't been able to offer me much sympathy as I am on the frontlines. I have friends I haven't talked to in twenty years crawling out of the woodwork, thinking about me, hoping that I'm safe, telling me they're praying for me. And when I talk and share stories with those people, never once do they put me down, diminish my feelings, or tell me to suck it up. And my close friends check up on me nearly every day!

I know the reason for that is twofold—because I tell you things you don't want to hear (like use the mouthpiece, dummies) and my continued pain at the front lines reminds you that your actions and choices have consequences.

The longer you believe in and listen to and vote for people who want to pretend science doesn't exist, the people who want you to just keep puffing into that bell end—it'll work eventually!—the longer you prolong this for me. Your daughter and sister. The sicker America gets, the more people die for no reason, and the longer I have to live my life treating them.

It really hurts knowing that neither of you can put two plus two together on that—or that if you can—you don't care.

And, actually, that's what's most painful. That both of you would rather be right—just keep blowing into that bell end! It'll work any day now!—for your value of right, than try to help me. Care for me. Protect me. Realize that science is science and opinions are opinions and there shouldn't be any crossover between the two.

So that's why I've pulled back from my relationships with the both of you over the past few months. Because it's just as if you had to deal with people who told you to blow into the bell end of the horn, and that that's what they were going to do, to your personal detriment, continually—yeah. You'd start to back slowly away, too.

It's really hard to want to hang out with people like that, no matter how much time and love you've invested in them. I'm sorry. (For what it's worth, I'm sure you feel the same about me—you probably feel I'm prickly, and I am, because it feels to me like you want me to die, heh.)

Every time I hear y'all say something about how "people need to live their lives" or "it'll only be a few more months" or whatever else

Fox is selling you that week—keep using the bell end! It works! Just give it long enough!—it depresses me to no end. Which you actually noticed, Mom. Remember when you messaged me, worried about how depressed I'd sounded? And I tried to explain all this to you, only much more messily?

Because, yeah, I'm hella freaking depressed right now. I've spent the last two weeks feeling suicidal. Don't worry: my husband knows, I'm taking care of myself—but that's another reason I've pulled back.

Because both of you seem to think that there's some acceptable number of casualties that're tolerable. And this is where my metaphor breaks down, because no one dies when you try to blow into the bell end of a French horn.

Neither of you seem to realize that the more people who get sick and die, the longer I have to do my job. For every group of elderly people that hang out and get each other sick at a casino—that rolls down to me. For every kid who goes back to school and gets his whole family sick—that rolls down to me. For every prison outbreak we have —that rolls down to me. Hell—there's a positive patient at my mother-in-law's memory ward now! We just found that out this past week! And if that spreads, it'll roll down to me—or some other poor nurse like me.

The longer we allow there to be preventable deaths, the longer my actual, real-to-me, I-mostly-enjoy-living-it life is in actual, real, danger.

I'm really aghast and saddened by how quickly the both of you are willing to write other people off statistically, as if their lives had no meaning just because you didn't know them personally. (And above and beyond the sheer number of deaths, the life-ruining complications that people who survive covid will have to live with and will somehow have to get insurance for.) It's really dark and callous and frankly frightening.

And it makes it hard not to listen to either of you two talk about this, with your conditional maths from your desks at home, without thinking that I, too, am an acceptable casualty. Or that the work I do, trying to keep my patients alive, has no value, because you've already written them off.

My brain really doesn't need that nonsense going on right now. It's got plenty of nonsense up in there of its own.

I don't know how our relationships work after this. I don't know how to keep compassionately loving you both, as I have tried to do my whole life, when your deliberate actions continue to cause me pain. I don't know that it's even mentally healthy for me right now to keep trying. I really have to protect myself at the moment, and surround myself with people who listen when I talk, who sympathize with me, who understand that my fears and concerns are rational, and who don't try to diminish those fears just because they make them uncomfortable.

I suspect y'all think I'm just some blubbering softhearted bag of emotions—and you're not wrong. To some degree, I am—but I would posit that's actually what makes me worth knowing. And there's plenty of other people in my life who see value in my softness, my kindness, and in me caring enough about other people to make sure that as many of us as possible get through this mess alive.

So yeah. I'm going to keep being me. I am, Mother—oddly, I know!—exactly the person who you raised me to be. Whipsmart, strong, funny, kind, and Christ-like—to everyone. Literally everybody. Which means I can't write off a single soul that didn't have to die, much less for someone shouting on TV that I should be breathing through the bell end of a French horn for the "economy!" Jesus Christ—I mean that, literally—like what would Jesus think if he came back now and looked around. He'd be all, "Wait, you're letting people die... for this? I kicked over moneylenders' tables... so that you could kill the elderly for the economy? Are you kidding me right now?"

I don't know why you can't see the value of the values that you (ironically) instilled in me anymore, but they're still there, ticking away, nonetheless.

If either of you want to yell at me after this, I don't want to really hear it, and I'm likely to block both of y'all for a bit, regardless, just to protect my own mental wellbeing, so if you do respond and I don't, that's why.

I still love you both. I'm sorry I'm your difficult daughter/sister. I wish things were easier on all of us right now (boy howdy, do I) but it is what it is.

7/18/20

I feel like most of my online arguments these days boil down to, "And just why are you okay with people dying, again?"

7/19/20

I don't know a single health care professional who enjoys their job right now.

7/20/2020—password protected journal

Y'all, being a nurse puts me in touch with other nurses everywhere (especially on Twitter) and a friend there sent me a screenshot they got from a nursing agency....

They're offering $5600/week for RNs in Palm Beach, FL.

That's fucked.

Not that there won't be people who go to cash in on that—and I'm so sure they're going to be earning that money—but a) that's probably three, maybe even four times what the local nurses make and b) in fucking Florida? If that's where cheap-ass Florida, of all places, is at, that desperately looking for staff, Jesus.

If they're that low on willing bodies that they have to offer that much... that doesn't bode well for other hotspots. Keep in mind, too, that that's like any other temp gig—the agency is making even more off of those RNs on top of that!

I don't begrudge anyone that kind of cash for this kind of danger, and I'm sure they'll work them like dogs when they get there—but I am worried about the trend that this implies.

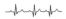

7/20/2020—password protected journal

Had two covid patients yesterday, both on high-flow O$_2$. One had already finished their course of remdesivir and had gotten convalescent plasma... and they were still on 90-100% O$_2$ all day long, with me going in and out and titrating things—I'm going to assume they got intubated overnight, alas.

The other was just starting their covid journey—and apparently their spouse was sick at home with it too. I know, because their kid called and was all, "Well, they haven't been tested, but they're already sick with it probably, so maybe they can visit because it won't matter?" and I was all, "Oh baby, no."

I think we were still at 16 patients housewide when I left; I forgot to check on my way out the door. (We are definitely lucky. So, so, so lucky.)

I've got a friend at work who is cashing in on covid so hardcore that he's going to quit his job with us and go and work in Arizona. Said he made $30,000 in one paycheck there, and I believe him. He's also the kind of crazy person who will work seven sixteen-hour shifts in a row, and once you get into doubletime....

Whereas our boss/hospital system is doing its darndest to save money by not authorizing any overtime, and one of the ways they're trying to combat that right now is by hiring nine new experienced RNs.

I was talking about that with my coworkers because, honestly, my boss is high if he thinks that's going to happen.

Yeah, we get paid well because we've got a good union, we're in the Bay Area, and California has staffing ratios.

But anyone who has experience and is mobile right now is likely going to be in a hotspot, cashing out, till they get burned out and then go chill someplace cheap for months on their earnings.

My boss is going to have a hard time finding people—with experience no less!—looking for new, real, long term positions, in the middle of all this nonsense.

Chad Wolf, acting DHS secretary under Trump, announces that he's going to travel across the country to put down BLM protests. (7/20/20)

7/20/20

So it's up to the states to mount their own covid responses, but for some reason when it comes to protests the response is nationalized?

7/21/20

Taking a two-hr. long "workplace violence prevention" class online, where I'm getting taught to do jujitsu, virtually, on angry patients.

Shoot me now? Please?

7/23/20

My intensivist just now, to a patient: "We just saved your life. Don't be a dick."

[CA: this patient was trying to hit us.]

7/29/20

Me, being in a bad mood today: I just...

[Dear husband]: Want the world to be a better place than it is. I know.

Me: Yeah. *Sigh*

(For what it's worth, this kind of quality telepathy is why we're married.)

Herman Cain dies of coronavirus, possibly contracted at a Trump rally. (7/30/20)

7/30/20

You know who I feel bad for?

Not Herman Cain—he made his bed.

No, I feel bad that MDs, RNs, RTs, janitors—probably hundreds of hospital staff, over the course of a month—who had to put themselves in personal danger of contracting covid to take care of Cain—FOR NOTHING.

It's one thing when my patients are unlucky, but man, can you imagine taking care of someone whose modus operandi for landing themselves in the hospital was active spite?

And hey, you know what I bet ALL OF HIS MEDICAL STAFF had in common in his room? THEY ALL WORE MASKS. Go figure!

7/30/20—personal journal

Had another bad panic attack today. Just the usual stuff, feeling absolutely helpless and overwhelmed. Accidentally timed it right so that my husband could stop what he was doing and come into the bedroom and just be a human weighted blanket till the worst of the crying passed. Took some Aleve, Ativan, and drank a Diet Coke (I needed the caffeine for my head) then took a two-hour nap.

I think I need to let go of some things. I'm just not sure what they are yet.

No rowing today. I've rowed or been at work every day for two weeks now. Figured my body could use a day off.

So could my brain, but I'm not sure how to find the off switch (other than the Ativan).

7/30/20

Profound words from my husband 15 mins ago: Dealing with the psychological ramifications of covid is a full-time job.

7/30/20

Tomorrow, no Twitter, just words and gardening. And a little rowing, as a treat.

AUGUST 2020

8/2/2020—password protected journal

Well, if members of my immediate family are data points, the US will continue to be screwed indefinitely, alas.
My folks just came back from their multistate road trip.
My brother just went to Turks and Caicos.
It's like they're not actually related to a nurse at all.

8/4/20

The longer I'm in isolation, the more my inside voice becomes my outside voice.

8/4/20

We've got an unknown critical intubated trauma patient here. They've been here for weeks, and in the charting under "patient preferences" one of my coworkers charted, "find identity."

And on a metaphorical level, I'm all, "Yeah, dude. Aren't we all?"

I'VE BEEN AVOIDING WRITING original material here for a while now. I mean, look, we're in August. It's been months.

Part of that is because I'm in a holding pattern right now over a holiday weekend (Memorial Day 2021), waiting to find out if my leave's been extended or not—my anxiety is through the roof, though I've been trying to manage it with medication and purposeful interactions with both my rowing machine and friends.

And part of it is just wondering... could I really go back to working bedside right now?

Would I be a good enough nurse?

Would I be safe?

And if the answer to either of those questions is no, well, then... who the hell am I?

A WRITER CAN ALWAYS WRITE. You don't even have to be putting pen to paper—you can look out the window and be writing in your head, because, to a large degree, being a writer is the experiential process of moving through the world as a person. It is akin to realizing everything in existence, from the sandwich you ate for lunch to the nostalgia you feel looking at old photos, has a thread attached, and that all you need to do is braid these threads into a story.

The sky is blue? Fantastic. What caliber of blue is it? Can—and should—you associate it with some other moment in your book? Is the sky as blue as the day your mother told you it was when you were born, or is it the same spitefully cheerful blue as the day she died?

What words can you use to describe its shade to your readers? Is it blue like cold ice, like waters deep enough to drown in, or your grandfather's glass eye? Which of these metaphors would mean more, depending on your book's theme and tone?

All you have to do to be a writer—to some degree—is want to write. And eventually, if you want this thing badly enough, if you think about how to do it, talk to other writers, read, and practice, you can do it and do it well.

Whereas being a nurse seems like it requires accoutrements.

You have to go to school. You cannot nurse without a doctor's permission. And I cannot "be" a nurse, looking out my window. I need the trappings of the hospital, the sterile walls, the cold beds, the beeping of an infinite number of alarms—and most of all, I need sick people. People who need me and who are tolerant of my care.

Writing I can do for merely myself, as I am now. (You, the future people who might read this book, are currently imaginary.) Whereas nursing is inherently interactive.

I cannot nurse from the safety of my couch.

So.

If I don't go back, does that part of me still exist? Is it baked in? Do I get credit for time served?

I don't really know.

I'm sure it seems all obvious to you, future-person-reading-this—I mean, yes, technically once a nurse, always a nurse, or some shit, right?

But you can't make me *feel* it, can you?

8/7/20

I want the "covid's just the flu" people to know we make fun of them every day as we leave work.

8/12/20

What'd you do during the pandemic, Cassie? Oh, you know, saved a few people's lives, and took a substantial amount of Ambien.

Yeah, I know it's probably long-term bad for me, brain-wise, but I don't have kids, so I don't really care.

I used to care, but now, fuck, if I get through this alive, what's a couple of lost brain cells? They're probably full of things I don't want to remember, anyhow.

8/14/20

One covid patient, and open for one admit in the next negative pressure room.

8/23/30—password protected journal

Got up this morning, rowed, gardened (during our brief moment of non-shitty air quality, California is on fire) and then my boss texted me at 10:30, seeing if I could come in....

And I did, like a sucker.

My hospital's totally full right now. It's bleak, and the ICU is out of ventilators. Nine covid patients in ICU, 17 housewide. I'm bummed, we'd been keeping the numbers down so well for so long.

My boss's text promised me no covid patients—I had to go down to PACU, though, because we've got four ICU patients down there in overflow.

Then I came home and watched Lovecraft Country, #noregrets, but I only wrote 800 words today on my breaks at work.

Hoping I can kick some ass tomorrow, though!

8/25/20

Just volunteered for OT at work.

Someone race over here and slap some sense into me.

No, really, I'm having a great shift. (In fact, I think I'm the only person having a great shift?) So I don't mind staying for four more hours today.

8/25/20

Tired and regretting all my life choices, but getting paid OT for them.

8/26/20

Home, showered, Ambiened.

Now to see if I can drag my sorry self out of bed in six hrs. to do it all again....

The coronavirus task force shoved a testing rule change through at the CDC while Dr. Fauci was under anesthesia for a non-covid related medical procedure. (8/26/20)

8/29/2020—personal journal

We're up to 20 covid patients housewide. Our most at one time yet. ICU had nine this past week, but now we're back to three.

So it goes.

SEPTEMBER 2020

9/7/20

It is so hot in my house right now that I'm actually going into work... for holiday pay, but also air conditioning!

9/12/20

I keep seeing shitty covid takes like, "when God wants me, I'll go, so why mask?" and honestly, if you're so willing to die when God wants you, do me a favor and never do any of the following:
  Go to the doctor
  Wear glasses/contacts
  Go to the dentist
  Work out at the gym
  Read books
  Wear makeup
  Drive a car

Go to school

Etc.

If you want to be just like God made you... then have at it. Abandon society and all its perks. But don't pretend God wants you to drive a stick shift more than he WANTS YOU AND OTHER PEOPLE TO NOT FREAKING DIE.

9/19/20

Bought myself many, many therapeutic plants tonight, instead of binging on ice cream. Feels like a small win. Actually, as I told a friend earlier, I think I mostly just shoved my feelings into the feelings hole.

Not sure how deep it goes or what happens when it's full, but hey.

The CDC pulls down language saying COVID aerisolizes.
(9/21/20)
[CA: this was terrifying at the time because it seemed the likely herald of a change in masking guidance.]

9/21/20

In hindsight, I really should've taken that Ativan, but now I feel it's too close to bedtime, so sure, let's just ride this panic attack out.

9/21/20

Pretty soon the CDC will just tell you to eat more GOYA beans.

[CA: for people who've forgotten, the dude who runs

GOYA was tight with Trump, and Trump posed with their cans of beans on his desk, which is an ethical violation.]

9/22/20

Did an extra ten hrs. for time and a half at work today. Got to hang out with a patient on the mend and we talked nothing but politics, and sometimes I really do like my job.

Oddly, my 70-year-old patient was able to do the math and realize that 200,000 covid deaths means that probably (conservatively?) 800,000 or almost a million American lives have been touched by covid, and that's just so far, and not counting ppl who didn't die.... Too bad the GOP can't do math.

Trump says covid "affects virtually nobody" at a campaign rally. (9/22/20)

9/22/20

My patients are not nobodies, asshole.

9/27/20

We're down to just five covid patients housewide here, halle-effing-lujah. I don't know if it'll hold, but it feels great.

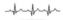

9/30/20

Remember when Ruth Bader Ginsburg died and you bought $$$ plants while on Ambien and now those chickens (err, plants) have come home to roost?

No? Just me?

I come in through the back door on workdays to strip in the laundry room. I'm glad this time I peeked out the front door to see plant-Christmas outside.

(In other news... massive unboxing tomorrow! The Amazon box has pumice and perlite in it!)

[CA: featured cat, Milly.]

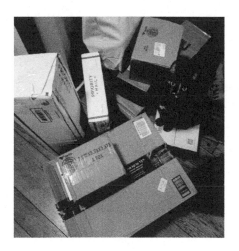

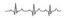

OCTOBER 2020

It gets leaked on Twitter that Trump has coronavirus.
(10/1/20)

10/1/20

TAKE SOME HCQ. ALL THE HCQ. TAKE IT NOW.

[CA: this is the abbreviation for the medication that Trump was shilling—hydroxychloroquine—that was useless for covid and actually dangerous unsupervised, if you'll recall. It killed a couple in Arizona who took a homemade version of it, and I personally may not have been shouting at the then-President in good faith.]

10/1/20

Slightly more cogently: It may make me a shitty person, but now that Trump reportedly has covid....

I want payback for every time I was scared to go into work

or into certain rooms. I want payback for crying helplessly as I told journalists my old hospital was out of PPE, as I desperately tried to get them supplies.

I want payback for having spent the entire month of July suicidal because everything felt so endless and no one gave a shit but me.

I want a refund on all the Ambien & Ativan I had to take to pretend to survive.

So he has it now?

After carelessly disregarding all science and health warnings and not just sitting idly by but actively discouraging public health and letting 200,000-plus people die, not caring what it meant to their families or how it'd break us at the hospital to attend to their deaths?

Good.

10/2/20

I just can't believe every single one of them thought they would be the one to beat science.

Trump doesn't wear PPE while healthcare workers are in the room with him at Walter Reed. (10/4/20)

10/5/20

Relatedly, I can't tell you how dismaying it is to stand outside a covid patient's room when that patient can talk and whatnot.

Part of you is all "hooray, they're getting better!"... but the rest of you is... damn, man, that's a lot of germs.

All of our covid patients on the mend in the ICU are

supposed to have masks on, which helps things, sure, but I just can't see Trump bothering to wear a mask indoors, no way, no how.

When I'm in a covid patient's room, I'm in full PPE. Does the WH staff have that available to them? Have they been fitted for n95s? Are they trained well enough to deal with this very literally life-threatening hazard?

I've always got a head covering on, goggles, apron, n95 mask. I never turn my back on a covid patient, I interact as little as possible with the room, and honestly, as little as possible, within my therapeutic boundaries, with the patient.

Luckily for me, our patients seem to get that. But does Trump? Or is he more like one of the patients we've been getting from a psych facility that's had an outbreak? Who can't help themselves from taking off their masks and coughing all the time?

My psych patients have an excuse, at least—what's his? And—I don't think the general public realizes how many layers of thought there are and how cautious, as health care providers, we are when dealing with this stuff.

Of course we are! It's our job!

But are they expecting housecleaners to obsessively change gloves, to never touch their masks with their bare hands, to think in that particular Battle Mode where every surface in the room—and also the goddamned air—is something that can attack you?

I mean, watch one donning-and-doffing video on YouTube. Is the staff of the WH legitimately prepared to do all that, 100% of the time, all the time? Consider too, back in the early days of covid, when [local hospital chain redacted] chose to do two things:

1) [They] had extra staff stand right outside of covid-positive patient rooms JUST TO WATCH NURSES DON AND

DOFF GEAR AND TELL THEM IF THEY DID IT WRONG. They paid someone. Just to watch them and make sure they did it safely!

2) [Redacted hospital] then told their staff that if they got covid, it wasn't [hospital's] fault for exposing them—because if they'd 'followed the rules' they never should've gotten it. They since recanted this, I hear. But yeah, those first few weeks in April, thrilling times!

I can 100% see the WH going that way—"Yo, we gave you a mask, it's not our fault you got sick!" And considering that he's in there trundling around, wiping his nose, coughing, touching everything with abandon and undoubtedly maskless —that's just a real dick move.

10/6/20

AND ALSO—I'm going to talk as much shit as I want about prominent GOP members catching covid because, EVEN IF I DO GET COVID, mine will have been hard earned, at work—not just out hating people, repealing rights, stealing money, killing the environment, etc.

Talking heads on Fox News say, "It's incredibly selfish of older people or neurotic people who are timid and afraid and won't come out of their basements to confine children and young people to miss out on the most important part of their lives." (10/6/20)
[CA, with heavy sarcasm: Yes. This one 'irreplaceable' October. No one will ever have an October again. Fucking murderers.]

A round this time in October, it became clear that America had no clear plan for or leadership initiative to deal with the upcoming holidays.

Literally every healthcare worker in America—four million of us nurses, and who knows how many other hospital staff—could see the wave beginning to crest, and could viscerally feel how unprepared we were. There was no cogent messaging and anytime anyone was rational about masks, the GOP undermined them.

We all knew that there was just going to be this great swamping wave of death.

I mean, hell, Fauci was barely able to control them, and even with him there the CDC kept moving goalposts, going so far as to freaking change their rules while he was in surgery!

Trump was still promising to pull a healthcare plan out of his ass —in fact the RNC said that his campaign ads were going to shift to focus on medically helping seniors—despite the fact that 95% of covid deaths were of people aged 50 or older—and... yeah.

We all knew there was no one we could trust to have our backs and there was no help coming.

10/22/20

I'm visiting my parents tomorrow, because I'm 100% two weeks out from my last covid patient at work now, and trying to figure out if I have the gumption to ask, and possibly find out, that they're voting for the man whose negligence could've killed me.

I love them, but I don't know how to deal with things. 2016 was disappointing enough, but after all this? Now? It's rough.

10/23/20

Woke up to a flat tire. No emotionally complicated trips today, so I'm going back to bed.

[CA: I still don't know who my parents voted for, if anyone, in 2020. I've never been able to stomach asking.]

10/23/20

Cancelled at work twice this week, suspect I'll be cancelled tomorrow (not enough patients, or personal seniority). Luckily, I can handle the pay hit, and the time off has been nice.

This is the longest "vacation" I've had off in years, but we can see the wave coming in T-minus three weeks.

10/24/20

Some nights I lie awake and wonder how any healthcare worker in the US could manage to come into work on 11/4 if Trump won. The tunnel feels long enough as it is.

If he wins, the tunnel will very clearly turn into the barrel of a gun.

Like, what would be the covid endgame in a second term? Fewer supplies, increased numbers of sicker patients, more long haulers who'll require rehab and care, and listening to people seriously talk about herd immunity like millions of people dying is okay, even in the abstract?

More shitty armchair scientists, more YouTube "PhDs," the shameful politicization of the CDC, less trust in the WHO? And deaths. So many deaths. For no real reason.

11/4 could be bad.

Because if Biden doesn't win it'll crush our souls before Trump gets the chance.

10/25/20

I have the kind of insomnia that stays up late, whereas my husband has the kind that gets up early.

That means this morning he read my Twitter thread about how much working in healthcare will suck if Trump wins, and he told me we'd figure out a way for me to quit, if so.

I already love him too much, in a possibly codependent fashion, and this is why.

He's amazing.

10/27/20

This is a note from one of my patients who couldn't have relatives in while we were going to compassionately extubate them and didn't know if they were going to survive long enough to get to hospice and die with family.

I sat there with them and we facetimed twenty people, near and far, because no one could come in due to covid visitation restrictions. So I read the scratchy notes they were writing for their loved ones. They weren't strong enough to hold them up, but they wanted everyone to know they loved them, and at the end they wrote a note for me. I blacked out my real name, but it says "Cassie = good!"

They actually survived long enough to go home and die with family.

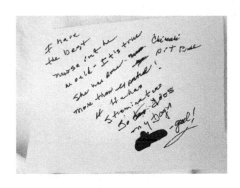

NOVEMBER 2020

11/2/20

Ladies, if a man tells you he believes in herd immunity, don't fuck him—that's the same kind of thinking that means he'll ditch you if you ever get cancer.

Whelp, if ever there were an Ambien night, it would be tonight. I'll be asleep in 20 mins, or I will have bought $200 worth of plants, or both!

11/3/20

The hazard of having been "the political nurse" is that my coworkers keep cruising by assuming I know shit, when I absolutely do not yet, lolsob.

God bless whoever put out the good-sized candy bars in the breakroom. I'm going to pound Snickers till we find out who is president.

11/3/20

We went from zero to three covid cases housewide here today, peeps. I really need the US to do right by us healthcare workers tonight.

I keep thinking about how the telepsych MD was asking a patient today, "Is anything important happening today?" And the patient was all, "Not that I can think of," and how blindingly jealous of them I was in that moment.

11/3/20

Also, a before-bed PSA: If you feel like you want to give up now, you're not alone. I know you're tired and it's been such a long road and justice seems just as far as grace.

Just try to stay spitefully alive for the next 12 hrs.

We can worry about the morning when we get there.

11/4/20

A patient's family wrote me a great note, which I showed management today, so I feel ok telling our GOP-conspiracy-believing respiratory therapist that he doesn't know how to fucking Google.

[CA: this was in regards to certain states being called for Biden.]

11/4/20

GOD HOW AM I STILL AT WORK TODAY? IT HAS BEEN A CENTURY.

11/5/20

Another day, another "trying to make sure the world bends towards justice" via the powers of my goddamned mind here.

If thoughts and prayers really worked, I'd have this shit on lock.

11/5/20

I can't believe that 70-some-odd million people voted for Covid.

Like   woooo-go-covid!-and-fuck-healthcare-workers-sideways! (That includes people from my own family.)

I'm relieved that adults will soon be in charge, but I'm aghast at the still-shooting-self-in-dick contingent here.

I'm >this< close to putting on a head lamp and stress gardening in the dark.

11/6/20—early AM

Don't ask how many plants I bought tonight. It was dark, there was Ambien, I ran out of ice cream, and it was a red devil dyckia. I mean come on, what choice did I have???

11/6/20—in the morning

What a way to wake up.

For once in a very long time, I actually mean it, God bless America.

11/6/20

Okay, so now that the election's over—I know it's early, but—let's all make a pact. Lean in.

You ready?

Don't travel for the holidays.

Don't you do it—and don't ask others to do it for you.

Covid hasn't gone away, and the situation on the ground is grim.

These next two months are going to be crucial for you and your loved ones' health. You need to stay home as much as possible. And (I'm sorry) no in person Thanksgiving and Christmas. I know. I'm a grinch who works every holiday, besides.

But the GOP was wrong (in this, as in so many other things) and covid is running amok in the midwest, hospitals are at capacity, brimming with the sickest of the sick, and when you add flu season on top of that, we're not going to be able to turn the tide on covid until Biden is in office Trump has made that ELABORATELY clear. The man gives no shits.

Our job is to survive until then, and to help one another to survive. And that means no holiday gatherings.

11/7/20

God. I'm not sure I can explain how good it feels to know that someone who gives a shit about covid and can implement real change is on the horizon.

All the other reasons too, obviously, but I feel like the firing squad stepped a football field back.

———

Early data from a large trial indicates that Covid-19 vaccine from Pfizer and BioNTech is strongly effective. (11/9/20)

———

11/9/20

Oh my gosh, this vaccine news is so heartening!!!!!

Everyone who volunteered for this vaccine trial is a legit hero.

The city of Tulsa is out of ICU beds. The city of El Paso is out of morgue space. The state of Iowa has beds but no staff. (11/9/20)

〜〜〜

11/9/2020—password protected journal

Okay, I'm about to put this in a header on the site here, but—**It has never been more important to socially isolate than it is right now.**

I have nurse contacts all over the US, and the situation on the ground is absolutely dreadful. A friend in the Midwest at a major level-one trauma center says they're pulling NICU nurses to work in med-surg units, going from exclusively taking care of babies to taking care of six adult patients, because they're running out of staff—and offering $500 per extra shift bonuses ON TOP of shift differential and overtime.

Hospitals in the US only speak the language of money, so please understand that if they're offering this, it's because their current staff is burnt out/on leave/quit—OR CURRENTLY SICK WITH COVID—and their pool of travelers has dwindled for the same reasons.

Hospitals in North Dakota are saying that asymptomatic covid nurses can keep working, taking care of covid patients—while ignoring the fact that many people who're asymptomatic become symptomatic AND that all of those nurses have to go on break somewhere, get gas somewhere, etc., WHILE FREAKING SHEDDING VIRUS.

The governor of Utah used the Emergency Broadcast System yesterday to get everyone's attention to tell them to mask up because their hospital system is at capacity.

Here's a tweet from another ICU nurse, talking about how they're using an extra 11 ICU RNS per shift [CA: see ancillary material]—she knows how lucky she is that her hospital is willing to pay for that extra staff, and that they're able to get that and use that. A lot of hospitals can't afford that and eventually (as the $500 shift bonus above indicates) you can't get blood from a stone.

Our ability to create beds out of nothingness is infinite—our ability to actually staff those beds is horribly, horribly finite. And every bed that has a covid patient in it—and these patients can require ICU care for two-three weeks apiece!—is one that can't take a flu or a heart attack or a stroke or a car accident trauma.

So—as a healthcare worker, and as someone who desperately wants everyone here to stay safe: **I implore you to re-enter lockdown conditions as much as you are able to locally.**

Consider that if your current local situation doesn't actually currently suck it is ONLY because you're in a state that has a mask mandate and your fellow humans are actually using them. Do not use this as an excuse to tempt goddamned fate.

And if you live in a state without a mask mandate, where people aren't taking this seriously—mask like your life depends on it and lock yourself down like you're on Alcatraz.

That's the only thing for it. I'm sorry. That's just how it is right now.

And don't even think about traveling for Thanksgiving or Christmas. Set expectations early. Repeat after me: "I'm staying home to protect my/your health because I love you. My concern for our health trumps gatherings this year."

People aren't going to want to hear this—I know, I'm getting shit from my own family. But that doesn't mean that it's not true.

You can't say, "Well, I've been good for six months"—covid doesn't care if you've earned points for prior lockdowns. It only cares about opportunities in the now. And if you look at the data, post one stinking motorcycle rally in Sturgis—or hell, the freaking White House—you'll realize that ANY cross-country trip right now is a BAD IDEA, as is associating with anyone indoors and/or maskless.

If we don't all do our best to starve it—absolutely starve it—of chances to get people sick, hospitals will continue to be over-whelmed, people who have non-covid problems won't receive care, and the deaths from covid and this umbrella of general fucked-uppery will continue to spread.

Don't do that to yourself, your conscience, your grandma, your kids, or me, your friendly neighborhood ICU RN.

Kansas City Metro reaches "uncontrolled community spread of covid." The state of Ohio is now low on ICU beds. (11/10/20)

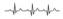

11/10/20

Y'all, I love you and if you've been following me for awhile, you know that my nurse-driven anxiety radar is about 2 weeks ahead of the national mood.

Go and get supplies now.

Prepare for lockdown. Even if things are OK near you. Just do it.

Trust me. Please. I want you to live.

11/10/20—tweet in response to another nurse saying she's quitting.

I'm not calling this nurse out in the least. I'm just saying that if the US continues to treat its health care workers like garbage, there will be a lot fewer of us in the coming months. Anyone who has options to go elsewhere will take them.

I love my job. I'd still leave it if I could.

11/10/20

That moment of extended existential dread after you beg people you know to do the right thing, even though it hasn't really worked in the past, and yet you still, out of love, cannot somehow stop trying.

11/11/20—email to my parents, after they decided to move cross-country.

Going into this, I just want you to know that this'll be my last email on the subject (she says, both because it's true, and because I hope that means that you'll bother to read it all.)

Mom, no amount of money is worth your life. I'll pay you your money back if the movers won't refund it.

Moving cross country during what is going to be the worst surge of a once-in-a-lifetime pandemic is ridiculous.

Nothing is going to get better in the next month or six weeks. Thanksgiving is going to hit the US like a car wreck. You will be travelling to Texas in December after the entire nation makes bad choices—entering an utterly unprecedented window during which there will be no beds available. None. No hospital beds. Even if you dodge covid, if you get sick, if you have a car wreck, if you get the flu, if you have another pulmonary embolism, you will be on a bed in a hospital hallway, alone—assuming they have hall beds available, at this rate. Assuming they don't have you in a tent somewhere. Or drive you three hours away to the next available hospital in an ambulance. You will be getting third-rate care from fourth-rate practitioners—and it won't be their fault. It's just that outpatient pediatricians will be the only staff left, the only ones who aren't burnt out, personally sick with covid, or taking care of family members that are. (I'm not even joking. The American healthcare system is run on hope and magic beans, and hospital emergency staff rosters are just not that deep.)

This is my last email on the subject, because I don't want to push you too far—but I also can't sit here in Dec-Jan (because it's not going to get any better. Christmas is just going to set off another round) knowing that I did not do my level best to make you see sense.

I need to sleep at night knowing I tried my hardest to keep you alive.

I would've said something earlier when I visited, if I had known how bad it was going to get. I'm sorry I didn't, but I had no idea then how bad the Midwest was becoming. I totally thought this move, while inherently dangerous because, duh, pandemic, was still somehow manageable, if you both tried your hardest to be safe. I cringed at the thought of you on a plane, but I thought, "Man, they'll be so much happier in Texas. I can suck it up."

And if, by some miracle, you could move RIGHT NOW THIS VERY MOMENT—I would still grit my teeth about the situation, but I would wave good-bye, because you might thread the needle and get there safely in time to hunker down and figure out a grocery delivery system. (Although looking at the hospital utilization graph I've attached, I'd still be really scared for you.)

But right now, the trajectory that the US is on, 8-12 weeks out? There's no way you can be safe, for two reasons:

1. you will be getting shitty care if you need to be hospitalized for literally any reason, covid or non, and
2. every single person you come into contact with is going to be a danger to you.

One out of every 87 people in South Dakota has covid right now. That's insane, and those ratios are creeping southward. That's how many people you see at once at a decent grocery store. Once you start hitting numbers like that you can't count on luck anymore, especially if these fools are maskless. It's like that old Palmolive commercial—at that point, you're soaking in it.

Okay.

That's it. That's my last impassioned plea. You don't even have to respond to this if you don't want to (unless you want me to make a check out to you or a moving company, and then I will SO FAST).

Like I said, I just have to be able to sleep at night.

With so much love,

Cassie

11/11/20—message to girls' chat

I know it's not going to work. And I know the fact that it's not going to work is going to hurt me. (In fact, right now, I just want to throw up.)

But I can't not try just one more time.

11/11/20

History will condemn Zuckerberg for allowing even one anti-mask Facebook group or meme to exist.

I'm essentially going to be an emergency broadcast system for the next 120-ish days.

(This is me announcing it and absolving myself so I won't even feel bad about yelling for the next four-six months.)

One in every 378 residents of the United States tests positive for covid. The seven-day average is 130,000, which is 71% more than the 54,000 of two weeks prior. Montana, Wisconsin, Oklahoma, Mississippi, Nebraska ICU beds running low. (11/12/20)

11/12/20

Can I just restate, for posterity, that Fox news is responsible for covid every bit as much as Trump is? And that Murdoch has an incalculable amount of blood on his hands? Thanks.

South Dakota has 2000 new cases in one day, and a 68.1% positivity rate. (11/12/20)

11/12/20

In case you're wondering how I'm handling covid data today, I just ate half a yellow cake with chocolate frosting.

11/13/20

My boomer parents, who have no actual reason nor need to move, have decided to put their house on the market right now, so they can move sometime in Dec/Jan, to Texas, when all this shit is cresting.

I've only been a nurse for 14 years, what the fuck do I know about anything?

11/13/2020—password protected journal

Hey so, sorry, I'm going to bang this drum one last time here (because I can't save my own parents, seemingly).

Please, please, please go out and get supplies right the fuck now and then hunker down.

The entire state of Iowa is out of staffed beds as of this morning. The city of Chicago and the state of New Mexico are going Shelter in Place from the 16-30th—other locations are SURE to follow.

There is a tsunami of death coming, not just from covid, but from our inability to care for anyone else in the system.

Be prepared, skip all of your Thanksgiving/Christmas plans, do not think of travelling until spring.

It just is what it is, okay? But don't you be a part of it if you don't have to.

11/15/2020—password protected journal

My parent's house sold in one day.

Now they're going to fly out to Texas and back to house shop, sometime in the next two weeks, and stay with my brother (who isn't masking and is going to the gym, I see on Instagram) and eventually move sometime at the end of Dec (assuming they don't get sick).

I tried, endlessly, so endlessly, to warn them.

BURN IT ALL DOWN.

11/15/20

The longer it takes Trump to leave, the higher the body count.

The state of Oklahoma is out of ICU beds. (11/15/20)

11/16/20

These series of tweets were in regard to the student loan debate coming up again, and someone saying that doctors should have their student loans abated, considering the current dangers of the hospital. I'm leaving it here because I think it'll help frame the staffing crisis coming up in December 2020.

Nurses need student loan relief too.

I've been a nurse long enough that I got my RN degree through my community college for $8000 total. I was on a waitlist for it back then, 15 years ago—I only got in because my school opened up a session starting spring semester.

Nowadays my coworkers are coming out of school, especially from private colleges if they want a degree faster, with $60-80,000 in student loans.

A secondary issue to this is credential creep.

I "only" have an associate's degree. I'm lucky enough that I've been bedside 14 years now and nursing is a field where experience trumps almost everything else—and I know I only want to be bedside (having left a desk job for this one).

But, just like anywhere, once you throw money in the mix and competitive schooling, there's plenty of people/groups/authorities that capitalize on this ability to shake future money-makers down.

The same whack letter organizations that have largely ABANDONED US DURING COVID—other than some sternly worded letters? *eyeroll*—like JACHO and ANCC, etc.—[CA: the Joint Commission on Healthcare Organizations and American Nurses Credentialing Center, respectively] want to make it so that everyone who is a nurse has to have an advanced degree.

Do you need that shit to be one?

FUCK NO.

(Am I biased? Possibly!)

With those advanced degrees oftentimes comes crippling debt with no actual bedside advantages and less physical experience. Maybe if you knew you wanted to go into management, you could use one, I guess.

But, by and large, requiring advanced degrees of nurses is a parasitic attempt to make money off of someone's future gains in a field that they might not even wind up liking, taking years away from bedside practical experience that would be more useful and profitable to them, long term.

You see this in every field (especially female- and POC-dominated ones, as nursing once was)—the banks and trade associations can't have you lady folk or "foreigners" make a reasonable wage without being penalized in other ways.

So they keep kicking the bar further down the field, while pretending that additional degrees (and lucrative/predatory student loans and colleges) are essential to public health and safety.

In any case—school should be free, and student loans should be abolished—and honestly, at the end of this, that's the literal LEAST you could do for healthcare workers of the now and the ones meant to replenish us in the future.

11/18/20

    We're up to nine covid cases housewide, four in the ICU, and one in a Rotoprone, which is mine and my student's.

    We also are stopping visitation again, as of tomorrow.

    [CA: A Rotoprone bed is a fancy bed for rotating people —it's an apparatus rather like a space-arm, and it grabs hold of the very-well-cushioned-patient and turns them upside down for you. It's also capable of rocking a patient back and forth, like a cradle, which helps mobilize secretions in their lungs, so we can try to suck them out with suction.]

11/18/2020—password protected journal

Back into the covid mines at work. Had a 70-plus woman with covid today.

    My parents are having home inspections and then weekend visitors coming down from Oregon, because of course they are.

    And then they're flying out to Texas on the 30th.

    The cognitive dissonance of talking to my 70-plus mom about all of her maskless plans after having watched someone her age circle the drain for twelve hours.... Well... it's a lot.

The Trump administration's vaccine distribution team confirms they have "no plans" of talking with President-elect Biden's vaccine distribution team. (11/19/20)

11/19/20

Whelp, we're full-up. And only five covid pts. Not sure where we'd put anymore, if any one of the positive patients on other floors crash.

My chirpy new traveler-trainee, earlier: Can I go down the hall?

Me, weary: Why?

New trainee: They're intubating a covid patient! Maybe I can help!

Me: Oh, no, baby. Come back from the woodchipper. Your turn will come, don't rush it.

11/19/20

I don't know why Republicans think the God they pray to, that's going to except them from covid, isn't the same God my patient's family is praying too right now, via facetime, as they hold their 3 yr old up to see their Grandma, while their Grandma is being held, medically paralyzed, on their left side at a 65 degree angle, in a specialty rotation bed, to maintain some semblance of lung function.

Either they're praying to two entirely different Jesus, or that GOP-Jesus is a fucker.

11/19/20

It's really frustrating to not have the right words to explain all this covid/nursing as someone who writes professionally.

When you're a writer you're used to thinking, "There's some perfect way to explain this experience. If I keep trying, I'll get it right, and people will understand me. I can make this experience universal. I can change lives."

I keep trying, and there's just... not. I feel like a whiner. We're merely full, but not slammed. But I can't help but see what's coming for us. And I feel how disposable our lives and the candlewicks of our souls seem to be.

I'm like so good at compartmentalizing now, y'all don't even have any idea. But I can't keep hoping that if I say the right thing once to the right person, somehow it'll change all this. Somehow it'll make other people care, make other people stop and think, and get the rest to mask.

I guess that's the stupid "American exceptionalism" happening in me, to I think that there could be an answer inside of me somewhere, that'd actually make a difference.

I guess that's good to have. That eight months of bullshit haven't beat it out.

It's just like a puzzle I can't put aside, though. Why don't people care? Why can't people care? Why don't people listen? How can I make them?

What else is there that I could possibly do to stave this thing off again?

But... there's nothing.

I can't even convince my own parents not to have visitors over this weekend. I can't even save them.

I feel like a failure, every single day.

I don't understand any of this, and I've made a semi-lucrative side-career out of distilling human experiences into words.

But for all this, for all the malignant ignorance, the harm we've done to our fellow humans, and are still doing every day... words fail me.

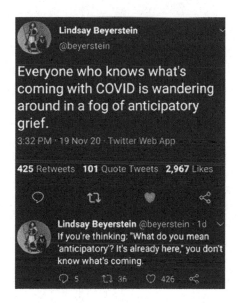

Lindsay Beyerstein
@beyerstein

Everyone who knows what's coming with COVID is wandering around in a fog of anticipatory grief.

3:32 PM · 19 Nov 20 · Twitter Web App

425 Retweets 101 Quote Tweets 2,967 Likes

Lindsay Beyerstein @beyerstein · 1d
If you're thinking: "What do you mean 'anticipatory'? It's already here," you don't know what's coming.

5   36   426

11/20/20—password protected journal

I think the real reason I've written so much this year is just the same reason I always write—to feel seen (and to a lesser degree, prove I exist).

And this year I've just needed to feel seen a whole hell of a lot more, heh.

I feel like everything now is just one long game of "the floor is lava!" at work until there's a vaccine out, you know?

I bought a ton of groceries earlier in the week and have every intention of just hunkering down until there's a vaccine and that's it. Everything—I mean everything—delivery. We subscribe to an organic veggie CSA and HelloFresh. I know we're lucky that we can afford it. Some part of that, though, is also me not wanting to interact with the world now that I'm working with covid patients again at work. It seems like if I can afford it, I ought to.

Anyhow, it'll just be work, the pharmacy, the gas station as needed, and that's it for the duration. I still feel like most healthcare workers who are getting infected are getting it via community spread rather than at work (because I don't know about them, but at work I'm hella zipped up). I'm still lucky though because in the ICU most people are intubated and on ventilators, which really limits spread opportunities, as the tube keeps the germs in.

11/21/2020—password protected journal

Y'ALL.

My hospital system is SO ON IT.

(By which I mean they ran the numbers and figured out that saving us is what will keep them profitable, lol.)

They're dropping a million bucks on ten of those fancy freezers—but they plug into the wall and can be driven around and run off of an inverter in a van, so they can transport them statewide—and we should be getting our first doses of the Pfizer vaccine by the end of December!!!

There is a light at the end of the tunnel. I can't believe it!

11/21/20

Today at work I facetimed a family who wanted to see their patriarch, who had had a stroke.

Ten people in a single room all talking and singing to the man they all love, knowing they may not get to see him again in person.

They all had masks on, even indoors.

It gave me hope.

The state of Nevada institutes a three-week statewide "pause."
(11/22/20)
Arizona ICUs are full. (11/23/20)

11/24/20—password protected journal

So I went to work today—we're up to 18 cases by the end of the day and half of them were in in ICU, and I had two of them(ish). The lady I had last week on the Rotoprone bed is on comfort care now and will probably be dead by midnight. Oddly, one of my patients from today had covid, but he's so far out from when he got it—he's been hospitalized since 10/25(!!!) that they'd discontinued isolation precautions on him because he shouldn't be able to transmit virus anymore.

That was cool/interesting/sad. I was happy to get to take some gear off, but at the same time, dude's been intubated and extubated FOUR TIMES. Kept getting better, going to the floor, and then tanking again and coming back to us. (He's in his 40s, BTW.) The last extubation was today. Hopefully it's the charm.

On the personal side, remember how my parents are moving to Texas in the middle of a pandemic because fuck me, science, and any current version of reality?

I message my mom today—they flew out yesterday—and she told me she's got a "bad cold that she caught from my dad."

AMAZEBALLS.

Just amazing.

I didn't know how to respond, honestly. I was at work. I wanted to cry. But like, what is there to do? (Did I mention here that because they were moving, a bunch of friends and relatives visited them last week, so my dad sent me a photo of six people over 70, indoors, several from out of town, with nary a mask between them?)

So like, if I call her up and give her shit and she's got it—well, there's nothing to do about it now, so what's the point?

If I make my dad feel like shit for giving it to her (while he likely still has it), what also is the point?

If she lives and learns no lessons—point?

If she gets hospitalized and/or worse—point?

There's no way to win.

I don't fucking know.

They're staying with my brother now, so I'm sure that's great too, in that he's not fond of masks, so either they're giving him stuff and/or possibly catching things from him (if they indeed have a cold and not worse).

Just FML, basically.

I'll call tomorrow and listen to her voice and see what that tells me.

Southern California is trying to dump patients on us too, BTW. Our head intensivist is all, "Yeah, fuck you, we don't want them," which is great, because we don't.

BUT ALSO: This past weekend's charge nurse tested positive for covid last night. (This past weekend that I very wisely decided to get call off for, knowing it would be the last lull we'd have for months.)

Turns out several other of my coworkers are out with it now too, which is why nightshift is dying for staff. Hopefully not literally. Yeehaw.

And now they've got signs up in the breakroom, saying no more than three people can be eating in there at a time. Yours truly has been eating in an abandoned waiting room for months, heh.

AND: Our management is ripping our hospital into pieces, intentionally.

Five different directors have been fired or have "retired" in the past month—including our own ICU director, and let me tell you how GOOD THAT FEELS RIGHT BEFORE A SURGE.

So we currently have no real boss, just an interim lady who means well but whose contract is up at the end of Dec.

My hospital's run by two unions, ours (the nurses) and the other one, comprised of respiratory therapists, all the lab techs, CT techs, x-ray techs, etc.

Anyhow—their contract was up earlier in the year—and management tried to fuck them in the neck. Management's opening salvo cancelled all of their retirements. Some of these RTs have worked for the hospital for 30-plus years.

Their current contract offering isn't much better, so they're all— literally every other service in the hospital other than nurses and doctors—going on strike shortly.

I don't blame them.

So yeah.

Parents possibly having covid feels great. Having worked in the recent past with coworkers who now have covid feels great. And knowing that my hospital administration is trying to fuck us sideways IN THE MIDDLE OF A SURGE also feels fan-fucking-tastic.

11/27/20

We need to bring back those old evangelical STD metaphors for covid, where they're actually applicable. "If you breath air with other people, it's like chewing their gum, and also the gum of everyone they've interacted with for the past 14 days. Do you want that?"

11/27/20

Y'all, it's been so hard to look at all these Black Friday deals in my inbox and ignore them. I usually have great self-control, but now I'm all, "Fuck it, I might die, so I really need 12 venus fly traps."

11/28/20

A sad thing I've been thinking about, and have decided to share, is how we're going into to the "Don't let Grandma die until after Christmas!" part of the year and how much that sucks, both for families and staff, given everything that's going down.

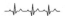

DECEMBER 2020

12/1/20

I've had the past week off (since Weds) and we went from six to 17 covid pts. Half are in the ICU (two of them are mine today).

12/2/20

Woke up from a nightmare about being in a plane and running out of fuel over open water.

    I managed to sleep some more, but then had a dream about taking nimodipine, so either I've got a subarachnoid hemorrhage or my brain would like me to be nicer to it today. I'm going to go garden.

2760 people reported dead in the United States from coron-
avirus on Wednesday, more than on any other day so far.
(12/2/20)

12/2/20

One of these was my patient from yesterday (and last week, and the week before that). It sucks.

(I should clarify: this is one death, only I took care of the patient for several weeks in a row, rather than three separate deaths.)

Not sure which is worse/better, though.

12/3/2020—password protected journal

S poke with my mother on the phone yesterday. It does indeed sound like she had a head cold—and then I was talking about precautions, and she was all, "Yes, but if I wear a mask, why isn't it safe to go out?" and I'm all, "Can you just not tempt fate? AND ALSO YOU GOT A HEAD COLD. Obviously your safety game is weak!" (only nicer, slightly.)

I can't believe we crested 3100 deaths a day here in the US.

12/4/20

Being a nurse this year feels like playing Dark Souls III in real life with no save points.

[CA: Dark Souls is a notoriously difficult video game.]

12/4/20—password protected journal

It's been a hard day to concentrate, really. I can feel the wheels falling off again inside my head, re: work and covid and people online and in the world still being maskless, anti-vax dumbasses.

Because I don't know that I'm strong enough to do all this again for a second time. It hurts so bad and it breaks my brain. I'm so angry one minute and then so indescribably sad the next—it's like my thoughts are treading water endlessly, with nothing ever to let them rest.

Some things are still good—my health, my husband, our relationship—but watching the upcoming unending wave of darkness, this tsunami on the horizon, just overwhelms any particular personal brightness.

And there's not even a point in trying to escape it because it just is. It's everywhere, and it's not going to go away, and it's going to take months and months. And people (who I am related to, even!) are still so terribly fucking, fucking dumb.

It's really hard to have empathy for everyone, and to some degree I don't want to anymore. I just want to hog it all for myself and people who listen. Being a good person fucking sucks (don't let anyone tell you otherwise). It sucks even when you're getting paid to do it. Maybe more, because you legit have buy in.

I've spent my whole life thinking about myself in one way—and then this year I had to walk through a tar pit, and I feel like it almost got me—and it took me months to put myself back together into this current version of me. New Cassie, Now with Dents!

And so just knowing more tar is coming, more endless stupidity, more dealing with the fallout of people's bad decisions, listening to people weep on facetime because they killed their grandma, having made decisions THEY DIDN'T HAVE TO MAKE because they were let down governmentally, systematically, educationally, by their churches, etc., is heartbreaking.

I don't know how I can do my job without feeling things, because that's not good for my brain—I can compartmentalize like a fucking mofo, but I know doing too much of that leads to disassociation, which is also very not good, because then I feel so distant from the world.

I always lowkey do that anyhow, but this just makes it so much worse. Between people not believing things on the internet, and just in general—I had this happen when I was a burn nurse. No one wanted to know what my job was, really, because it was gross and frightening. It was just my burden to bear, solo, and I got used to it.

But at the same time—I never had to see anyone wander around outdoors with lit matches, you know?

I was OK holding things in back then, when it was just a pact between me and the patients and my coworkers. But now that I see people wander around in society, trying to, looking to, going to get, burned (metaphorically) by this—it's really fucking hard.

(And in my darker moments, it makes me want to grab their faces and curb them against the pavement, which is not a very nursely thought at all. I don't enjoy being a violent person on the inside. I'm so angry, y'all. There's so much rage in me. I want to quench it, but to be honest I don't know if it's safe to do that. What if that's the only thing holding me together, keeping me putting one foot after the next, just sheer fucking spite?)

Anyhow. I'm trying to stay connected right now, really. I know the drill: people, gardening, exercise.

But this is just a lot, on all fronts. It just is.

My husband keeps telling me to go to therapy, but here's the thing about that—I never once needed therapy as a burn nurse, for being a burn nurse, because I had that shit on lock. For being a morbidly depressed author? Oh yes. But never work related, heh.

If I hadn't, though—what would've been my ethical responsibility there? Because I can close my eyes and conjure up shit that would make you puke on your shoes. If I couldn't have hacked that, if I needed to share that with someone else—what civilian could I have ever expected to help?

It wouldn't have been ethical of me to give that shit to someone else's brain.

And that's how I feel about covid now, too.

It'd be different if I saw a therapist who lived on Mars, I guess, who wouldn't also be participating in this society. But, obviously by default, any current therapist would—and I don't know what they're going through. I don't want to spew shit out at someone who may very well have lost, or be going to lose a relative, and scarring them too.

That's not right.

I don't even know what I'd say to them anyways.

"Hi, yes, I've been epically betrayed by my country in general and my relatives in particular and there's Not Anything I Can Do."

"Yes, I think I have PTSD. No, I manage it pretty well casually, thanks."

What would even be the point?

All this shit is situational, and realizing that is the only leverage on my brain that I've got—and I don't need a therapist to tell me that.

I just have to tough it through, again. Despite the fact that round one almost broke me. Getting the vaccine will help. Watching people die who didn't have to, well....

I hope I like the new version of me, the one I'll get to be on the other side of all this. She's going to be tougher and more distant and more weird and have an even harder time being present, and people are going to talk to her in the future and be all, "Wow, that must have been so hard for you" and she'll get to smile tightly at them and say, "Why, yes, yes it was," because that's what people who move in polite societies do.

Eh, it'll all fit in a box again someday.

Just have to keep getting bigger boxes to shove things in, is all.

And make sure I don't fall in myself.

12/5/20

I volunteered to stay till 11 PM. Someone come and slap my goodwill out of my head.

12/6/20

The sheer exuberant joy my coworkers and I feel when any member of the Trump administration contracts covid is unparalleled.

To quote a friend, "I hope they intubate him without sedation."

12/6/20

Paralyzing another covid patient to maintain their lung function.

12/7/20—text from work—this is the majority of our floors.

Mon, Dec 7, 2020 10:02 PM

Staffing Help Needed
Hi All;
We are having a surge of patients and need nurses in ICU (2-3), 4th, 5th, and 6th floor. Please call staffing if you can help. Thank you so much! Sorry for the late notice, it has been a quickly evolving situation.
Reply with YES to confirm receipt or

Trump administration passed on securing additional Pfizer doses "months ago." (12/7/20)

First Pfizer vaccine given to a 90-year-old woman in England.
(12/8/20)

12/8/20

Lord, please, by the end of this may I not become a professional angry lady, as I prefer just to maintain my high-ranked-yet-amateur status for my heart condition. Thank you.

12/8/20

These fools want you to die.
> For real.
> It's their only interest in life.
> It's what they jack off to at night.
> Don't listen to them.

THAT LAST TWEET was in response to Jim Jordan, who related the WHO recommending not hugging over the holidays to the inability to say "Merry Christmas" LIKE ANYONE GIVES A FUCK.

NEWSFLASH: NO ONE IS COMING FOR CHRISTMAS!

Look deep into your heart, members of the GOP.

DO YOU HONESTLY THINK PEOPLE DON'T WANT TO TAKE A HOLIDAY BREAK?

Everyone loves holidays!

Everyone loves Christmas!

I'm sorry that you think that the baby Jesus isn't super involved in Christmas anymore, but UNTIL I SEE YOU GIVING A SHIT ABOUT HIM LITERALLY ANY OTHER FUCKING DAY OF THE FUCKING YEAR WHILE PEOPLE ARE DYING THEN FUCK YOU.

. . .

I ASK YOU AGAIN.

WHY DOES YOUR VERSION OF JESUS WANT PEOPLE TO DIE?

I GOT SO tired of hearing about God last year y'all.

Tired in my BONES.

People are at the hospital desperately wanting miracles for loved ones, while on TV pastors and the President pushed to meet in person, pretending like their "religious liberties" outweigh the needs of the community in THE MIDDLE OF A GODDAMNED PLAGUE, because they needed their collection plates full.

Because that's all it is/was.

They just wanted your money.

Needed the coffers to keep flowing, to pay for those fancy shoes and those private planes.

Honestly, you, as a parishioner—do you think your God is so small that he doesn't recognize your prayers at home, one on one? Do you think that if He can't hear your choir then He forgets His name if you all aren't all together, singing it?

Do you think that maybe He can give you a pass during a FUCKING PLAGUE YEAR?

AND IF YOU'RE rocking back saying, "Well, God knows when it's my time," then please again, go fuck yourself and never avail yourself of modern medical care, anything in your medicine cabinet, or any medical advice you've ever received.

"God knows when it's my time," says the wealthy person with

access to health care who isn't in danger of giving covid to anyone else, while on adequate blood pressure medication.

Because I was there when plenty of people WHO DIDN'T WANT TO GO SEE JESUS died, and for some reason NONE OF THEM NOR THEIR FAMILES FOUND PEACE IN IT.

You know why?

Because none of this had to happen!

N O N E.

So when you say, "God knows when it's my time," in relation to last year and covid, it's like spitting on half a million graves.

Let's flip your statement.

Did those people deserve to die? Because they had to serve you food in restaurants or bag your groceries? Was God all, "Yeah, let me kill Blacks and Latinos and Indigenous people in vastly higher quantities because I'm a fucking dick"?

Is that your God?

I'm not religious anymore (I don't know if you could tell, heh.)

I used to be, though. A lot. I was a true believer, the kind of super-fun kid who told other kids at the slumber parties that they were probably going to hell.

But the more I moved in the world and thought about things, the harder believing became.

We're all probably familiar with the Problem of Evil—i.e., if God truly is God, why does evil exist in the world? And if God allows evil to exist... doesn't that make him an asshole?

I was never able to reconcile those things inside my head, and I decided that the easier route was believing that God wasn't there. (With a side of, "If God is there, and me being a covid-nurse doesn't get me into Heaven later, then fuck him.")

I know, however, that believers would say that that gap between is where faith comes in. The whole "let go and let God" thing, where you let "Jesus take the wheel" and believe that "everything happens for a reason."

And while there is a psychological benefit in acknowledging that certain events are out of your control and you are unable to change them—indeed, we are each only capable of changing our own minds, truly, no matter how hard we try otherwise—I'm not okay with just "giving up."

Because statements like that absolve the person believing them or saying them of personal responsibility and are used, in their most essential form, to justify suffering.

Suffering is not noble.

Let me repeat: Suffering is not noble.

You can find meaning in suffering, yes, and suffering can change you, definitely, but suffering, in and of itself, should not be a goal. Not for yourself, not for anyone.

We want to mythologize pain because we long for stories—fictional, and personal—to have meaning, and we want to feel like we've conquered something along the way.

But if you start believing that suffering is noble, then it becomes okay to sit back and watch people suffer on some level. You see that, right? You begin to believe that people "need" to hurt... to... what? Grow up? To further experience capitalism? *Fuck.*

Look, you can see this now, with the student loan debates.

How amazing would it be for a huge segment of the US, the one that's got student loan debt wrapped around its neck like a yoke, to suddenly be free? What magnificent changes could that create in opportunities, and how would freeing up all those (priorly personally useless to the debtor) payments flood the economy?

But any time this comes up, some shriveled soul says, "Let's not be too hasty! I paid my student loans! Everyone else should have to pay theirs as well, or it's unfair to me!"

Well let's flip that lens, too:

Say a miraculous new drug for cancer comes out, something that can cure all cancers, everywhere, all the time.

Would former cancer patients say, "Let's not be too hasty!" do you think?

No, because former cancer patients usually aren't assholes.

But what's the difference between former cancer patients and student-loan-forgiveness-haters?

Former cancer patients know that suffering isn't noble.

Their suffering was not an abstract thing like a dollar amount (except for all the times it likely, very expensively, was, alas. I'm glad that GoFundMes exist, even as I am horrified by the fact that they must.) Cancer survivors' suffering was something that permutated their entire body, eating at their cells, and they longed to be rid of it.

Whereas the student-loan-forgiveness-haters have mythologized their suffering. They "overcame!" their student loan debt, and it put hair on their chest and made them into the men and women they are today, allegedly. Thus, no one else can be expected to "skip the line" and everyone should be forced to suffer equally.

But... why?

I'm honestly asking.

Why?

If you start telling me that it is good for people to work, I heartily agree with you. But then, how come certain jobs aren't expected to pay a living wage, despite the fact that they are full time? And still I ask, why? A job in food services or janitorial shouldn't be considered punishment, should it? Just because it may not be a job that you want, that doesn't mean that it isn't still a job that should be treated with decent pay and respect.

Can you explain to me, in a non-punitive way, why certain people should not be able to: eat, have healthcare, get education, and find adequate shelter?

I can explain to you how come people lack those things—because the social safety net has been eroded, the ACA has been eroded, etc.

But... why?

Why don't we make sure everyone has enough to eat? Why don't we keep on top of preventative care, and why didn't we give people a universal basic income to keep them safe inside during covid to save lives?

It is because of (and was because of) Jordan and his ilk.

The kind of people who go to church every Sunday, who sing the songs and listen to the pulpits, but who let the true word of God flow through them, like the water in the center of a river, never touching either bank.

It's because if you give stuff up to God, it neatly becomes somebody else's problem.

And I guess God'll get to it when he gets the chance.

More than a third of Americans live in areas where hospitals are critically short of ICU beds. (12/9/20)

12/9/20

When they eventually make a documentary about all this— one of several, I'm sure—some documentary is going to source out everyone in @fmanjoo's purported Thanksgiving covid bubble, and it's going to make the *Law and Order* sound as the word THANKSGIVING fills the screen.

IN HINDSIGHT, this was around the time when I started giving no shits.

(I know, you're reading that, and thinking, nah, that was clearly sixty pages ago, BUT NO. Significantly fewer shits are given from here on out!)

I was so tired of watching people slowly die and exhausted by the world that I went in all guns blazing, all the time.

Farhad Manjoo, an NYT opinion guy, was the author of a pre-Thanksgiving piece that said essentially, "Yeah, covid's bad, but fuck it, I'm going to travel anyways," and then wrote a subsequent piece saying, "Gee, everyone's mental health is really bad right now, I wonder why?" as if there was NO CORRELATION BETWEEN THOSE EVENTS.

I couldn't stand it, that someone with that broad of audience was giving SUCH SHIT ADVICE and then being performatively naive on the far side. Which lead to me tweeting this on 12/9/20:

Hello, I would like to write an article for a national newspaper about All Of This, as an ICU RN. I'm a professional author and I promise I can turn in anywhere from 500-5000 words without cursing in real life (unlike on here).

That, in turn, led me to creating the Two Nurses Talking newsletter with another nurse friend of mine, where we talked about whatever we wanted to and cussed pretty much all of the time.

12/11/20

Woke up from a dream where I couldn't hug anyone and they all gave me shit about it, so that's fun.

Considering the greater incidence of covid among Black and Latino populations, white people not wearing a mask is a racist act of aggression.

12/11/20—excerpts from Two Nurses Talking's "soft" launch.

White People Not Wearing Masks is An Act of Racist Aggression

I MEANT WHAT I SAID, and I said it because it's true. (So much for the soft launch, let's just dig right in here!)

I'm writing this right now from my car in the Safeway parking lot near me, waiting for a prescription to be filled. I live in Oakland, CA, and my Safeway is on Fruitvale Ave, the same Fruitvale you may remember from the amazing and sad and anger-inducing movie *Fruitvale Station* that came out awhile back.

Many of my co-shoppers—if not the majority—are Black.

The only time I've ever come to blows in RL with someone who didn't have a mask on (not online, heh; online y'all know I'm always ready to brawl, for better or worse) was at this self-same grocery store a few weeks ago.

There was a white chick in an aisle with no mask on.

I lost my damn mind.

Well, first, I almost had a panic attack. Then I offered her a mask, and then when she didn't want to take one, said she "didn't need one"—I made a scene and told her "I see people die at work!"

It probably wasn't the sanest look, alas, but by then I really was having a panic attack. I told security about her, and they checked in, but apparently they're not allowed to make people leave. So then I called store management, who told me that they wanted everyone to wear masks, but that they couldn't enforce it on the ground, because people were unsafe, and they didn't want to put their employees in danger.

The irony of this, when that maskless woman was literally putting everyone in the entire store danger, is not lost on me.

In hindsight, I went about that all wrong.

I wish I'd had an edit button for that whole experience there—the kind I have here, writing this, slightly more calmly now.

I wish I'd been able to tell her—every time a white person doesn't wear a mask, they're putting Black people at risk and you're in the goddamned Black grocery store, woman. She looked like the kind of anti-science-yet-still-liberal-hippie-who-thinks-they're-an-ally   that that might have worked on.

AND EVERY SINGLE WORD OF IT WOULD'VE BEEN TRUE.

Black people are being so disproportionately punished right now in this pandemic, as are people of any other non-Caucasian ethnicity. And frankly (albeit non-scientifically), it's mostly white people spouting that, "but 99% of people are fine!" bullshit on Twitter, judging by profile photos. We'll get into the science of why that's a fucking lie later.

NEWSFLASH: 1 in 800 BLACK AMERICANS HAVE DIED FROM COVID. And indigenous people are getting crushed even harder!

So every time some white politician comes up in my feed on Twitter, and they're all, "What's next?!?! Cancelling Christmas?!?!?"—or in your family! Or on your Facebook! –

I want you to respond: YOU KNOW WHAT CANCELS CHRISTMAS OTHER PEOPLE'S CHRISTMASES PRETTY FUCKING, FAST?

KILLING GRANDMA.

And consider that the GRANDMA YOU KILL MAY NOT BE YOUR OWN.

Only white people are doing dumb shit like having massive Christmas parties.

Here's noted "Christian" Dave Ramsey, plunging ahead with his in-person monstrosity.

He's on record as saying, "Fear is not a fruit of the spirit."

FUUUUUUCCCCKKKK YOUUUUUUUUUUUUUU.

Dave Ramsey, I'm calling you out on this shit.

DO YOU KNOW WHAT MOST PEOPLE WHO HAVE

FAMILY MEMBERS INSIDE OF THE HOSPITAL GET TO DO, DAVE?

PRAY.

That's all they do.

Man, I've heard rosary prayers on facetime so much I could do them my goddamn self.

You're saying that people who get covid get to die because they didn't have enough faith and God didn't love them?

FUCK YOU FROM THE BOTTOM OF MY SOUL.

COMPLETELY.

You are a scabrous human being and I wish karma were real and you got what you deserved for that.

I weep to think that people like him get to call themselves Christians. Not only is he putting people who attend his function in danger, he's going to expose countless other people to danger as well —caterers, cleaners—and every one of those people who're "essential" to his party are likely in a lower socioeconomic bracket than he is, and if they do get sick, exposed to his maskless masses, they're unlikely to be able to afford his "skip the line" quality of care, and they'll be putting even more burden on whatever hospital system they're nearby!

I feel like every single time there's an event like this, there needs to be concomitant contact tracing immediately afterwards to see who bears the brunt of this idiocy.

It's almost always going to be non-white people, or the elderly, or both.

Real Christian look there, Dave, killing someone else's grandma. I hope you're fucking happy.

One more quick example of racism in action related to medical stuff before I call it quits today: Dr. Cleavon MD got asked to not go into a shift in Yuma Arizona because he's been preaching about ICU capacity and calling the governor of AZ out on his "we've still got beds!" shit for the past two weeks.

THIS IS THE SAME DOCTOR THAT PRESIDENT

BIDEN JUST CALLED UP A FEW DAYS AGO TO SAY THANKS FOR DOING GOOD WORK.

Why was he fired? Well, apart from the fact that he was causing a hospital system problems, could it have been because he was Black?

Very dang likely. Medicine is (like most professions, still, to this day!) racist, alas. It's everyone's job in medicine to break down these barriers and speak truth to power, BUT ESPECIALLY US WHITE PEOPLE.

Because people still want to discount the truth of Black and brown people's stories.

I am a white person. I may make fucking mistakes here (as we go along) and I'm 100% cool with being called out on them.

But also as a white person, I'm well aware I've got privilege and because of it I have an obligation to shout out racist stuff when I see it, because (for whatever shitty reason) white people might be able to listen to me more than when the person telling them is Black.

So—yeah. I'm telling you that white people not wearing masks is racist and I encourage you to pass it along.

(Back to a, uh, soft launch, lol, starting 12/16—subscribe if you're interested and tell your friends.)

– Cassie

[CA: Dr. Cleavon was rehired a day later after national outrage.]

Governor Newsom announces that the first truck of Pfizer has left Michigan for California. (12/13/20)

12/13/20

I want it to be public knowledge which of our politicians have gotten vaccinated. Live time. As it happens. Because I don't want a single one of those GOP effers to secretly get the shot and then talk smack about covid and its effects.

They're bad enough about being homophobic while being secretly gay, etc. I don't want any secret anti-science Tea Party no-masking politicians falling thru the cracks. I don't mind them getting the vax, but if they lie about covid's effects afterwards, I want them underground.

Texas ICU bed availability is at its lowest since the start of the pandemic. (12/14/20)

Trump White House Chief Security officer has to run a GoFundMe after leg amputation from covid. (12/14/20)

12/15/20

My great-aunt has been in a local ED since 11:30 last night with covid and a UTI. She was living with Alzheimer's at a nursing home. My cousins are going to let her pass.

I was wondering when this would strike home personally, and here we are.

She was a good woman.

12/15/20

Just got an email from work. Five intubations today. They're requesting we pre-staff up four or five RNs a shift from now thru Christmas.

12/16/20

Nothing like waking up to an email that says that your shift is four nurses short.

12/16/20—Two Nurses Talking newsletter excerpt

Covid RN PTSD

I don't want people to look at me strangely, but I also don't want to not tell you how it is.

I have a (mostly) private journal that I write my thoughts and feelings down in sometimes, as I have them, and that's important because, other than anger, I don't often let myself have feelings anymore, because I've perfected the art of disassociating.

People who know me know my brain is full of boxes. Cluttered with them, in fact, and that's where I put everything. Because when you're a nurse you're always expected to move on and perform—and far, far, far more so in times like these.

The downside of it is the general disconnect from humanity (which isn't great when taking care of humanity is your job) and the feeling of being unmoored. But if to be connected is to feel pain and not be able to function when people need me the most, well... that's why I journal.

To remember what it was like to get to have feelings, while they last.

I tell people astoundingly sad things sometimes, and then they come back a week later and they're all, "Hey, so, how are you?" in that gentle kind way where they're worried you'll break—and truth be told, I've completely forgotten. (Or I've seen so much sad stuff in the interim, I'm all, "Uh, you're going to have to be more specific, please.")

It's not like those feelings weren't legitimate in the moment. I did feel them, and I needed to express them (verbally, or in my journal) but I've just gotten so (cripplingly?) used to moving on.

Because not moving on isn't good for me—if I dwell, I get more depressed.

At the same time, though, when all you're doing is moving on—I don't know if that's healthy, good, or right, either.

Is it?

It is functional. Yes. But I feel like vast parts of my psyche are spring-loaded traps that I'll get to discover later. Maybe all these boxes I have are turning into jack-in-the-boxes, I don't know. I don't feel as whole as I did before all of this started, or perhaps even as whole as yesterday. When you run through all your memories with a melon-scooper, sometimes you have to really conscientiously try to be a person again afterwards. I don't want to be your strange friend who can do a human dance with dead eyes. But I don't want you to feel bad for me either, because that's strange too, and I know personally so many other people who have it worse and who need your pity more.

So yeah. I'm okay, mostly, as long as I've got enough cardboard and packing tape.

(It's just some days I'm not sure I really know what the word "okay" means.)

—Cassie

12/16/20

We've got 30-plus covid patients now. Today is pretty crazy.

I filled out my paperwork for the vaccine—no word on when, though.

12/16/20

When you're happily rocking out in isolation gear in your medically paralyzed covid patient's room to the Spotify playlist you made for your current book.... And NIN's "Fuck Me Like an Animal" comes on.

12/16/20

Oncoming nightshift intensivist: I feel like you all are offering me the last ticket for the Titanic.

12/16/2

My poor coworker, who went from having a fresh admit shit the bed with blood, into emergency intubation, central line placement, a massive transfusion and (unfortunately) a transfusion reaction, bedside EGD, trip to CT, and ultimately down to interventional radiology, just texted me thanks for helping her. :D

Every hour, two people in LA County die of covid. Nationally, 3611 people die of covid today.

Pfizer shipments are being held up, awaiting orders from the Trump administration. (12/16/20)

12/17/20

40-plus patients with covid now, house-wide.

12/17/20

Email from management—VAX IS IN HOUSE

Southern California is out of ICU beds. (12/17/20)

12/17/20—Two Nurses Talking newsletter

HOW ICU CAPACITY WORKS—JESUS CHRIST IT IS NOT THAT HARD TO UNDERSTAND, AKA THE ICU IS YOUR LAST STOP BETWEEN HEAVEN AND HELL

HEY THERE, ICU RN Cassie here. Let's break down how ICU capacity works and what affects it, m'kay?

BECAUSE I AM SEEING THINGS ON TWITTER THAT MAKE ME WANT TO STRANGLE PEOPLE.

I'm usually brusque with idiots, but this is a very special late night "I've worked two very long 12-hr-shifts and have another long-ass 12 to look forward to tomorrow," so there's going to be extra curse with curse-sauce.

People keep saying, "Oh look, the numbers are fluctuating" or, "Can't we bring in a Navy med boat?" or, "Why aren't they building tents?"

Here's the FIRST THING TO UNDERSTAND:

Hotels have beds!

Beds are not the problem here!

The problem is STAFFING THE BEDS.

When you talk about ICU capacity what you're really talking about is STAFF.

Someone (who meant well) was asking me on Twitter today why we can't just press gang people into helping with covid patients, á la women going into factory work during WWII while the menfolk were off at the front.

But that's a really shitty analogy when it comes to ICU capacity.

I'm not in isolation gear for 12 hrs. a day pounding rivets into steel, man.

I'm saving fucking lives. Trying to.

So a more apt comparison is ICU RNs to the fighter pilots. I've got roughly the same education as one (at least 5 years to become an RN, and that's without a bachelors) and I have to know JUST AS MUCH SHIT, and arguably what I do is just as expensive because what's more precious than a human life? And y'all know how much they charge for things at the hospital, heh.

You cannot just shake a tree and knock more ICU RNs out of it. Nor respiratory therapists! Or doctors! Or nurse practitioners!

I hope by now people aren't buying the whole "but it's just a flu season!" canard that Tucker Carlson would have you believe, 'cause it ain't. Yes though, in a typical flu season, we can get up to 100% full, and hey, you know, off season, someone hits a bus full of nuns or whatever, shit happens.

But the current problem is that:

A) EVERYWHERE IS FULL. There's no one we can call for reinforcements! We can't send extra patients to Southern California, nor can they send their extra patients up to us. THERE IS NO ROOM AT THE INN.

B) USUALLY, we use traveler RNs as stopgaps in these situations. But right now—THE ENTIRE NATION NEEDS TRAVELER NURSES.

I'm hearing stories of travelers getting $8000/week pay! That's utterly unheard of in normal times! (Not that they don't deserve it; they're working their asses off! Much love to my traveler RNs; get that money honey.)

· · ·

C) NORMAL STAFF nurses are quitting jobs they currently have to cash the fuck out.

Can you blame them?

We fucking watched maskless fools parade about in our faces for the past goddamned nine months.

If I worked in a place where I was going to get intentionally coughed on or assaulted in the grocery store for wearing scrubs, you'd best believe I'm going to get PAID THE FUCK OUT FOR IT. What loyalty would I have to a city that allowed parades of maskless people out and about? (What's, that Huntington Beach? Am I looking at you? WHY YES I AM you fucking armpit full of yahoos.)

D) NURSES ARE GETTING sick or having relatives of theirs get sick, who then require care and they themselves need to be out.

I've got a stepdown nurse who we've been training up to be an ICU nurse—two of her relatives have covid right now. She didn't have to quarantine because she didn't live with them, but it's happening to tons of nurses everywhere. And as long as we're still forced to participate in a non-lockdown, masks-optional society because of capitalism and poor governmental planning, this will continue....

E) COVID PATIENTS stay hospitalized (in those precious beds) longer.

A typical ICU stay is five-seven days. 14 days on the outside.

You want to know why?

Because that's about how long you can have a breathing tube in normally before you start to risk mouth-throat erosion. (Yes, we've all seen people be vented for up to three weeks; other nurses, don't you dare get pedantic with me right now.)

USUALLY though, we know whether or not you're going to die well before that—but if you're still on ventilator at 10-12 days and we can't get you off for non-covid reasons, we're going to need your family to shit or get off the pot: we're involving palliative care because chances are we're going to compassionately let you go or we're going to trach and PEG you (give you a tracheostomy to breathe through and a tube into your stomach for feeds) and downgrade you to another floor or send you to a skilled nursing facility for rehab.

But covid's a little different because it can rollercoaster you.

I took care of a guy two weeks ago who had been in our hospital since October and in the ICU for half of that

He got better, got downgraded to the step-down floor, got worse, got reintubated and back to ICU. Got better, went down again, got worse, got reintubated and ICU. Got better—you get the picture, right? He had been hospitalized (when I had him) for over 45 days, and at least half of those were in the ICU.

He wound up getting better! And leaving! (Miraculously enough.) But he ate up an ICU bed for at least 25 days!

And again—he survived! So it was all worth doing!

I'm not saying that's normal, but when your grandma comes in and has a stroke, we're not pussyfooting about her chances of living past day 10 all that often, my friend.

Whereas with covid, sometimes, yeah.

F) COMPLEXITY OF CARE:

So this goes back to the fighter pilot vs. riveters, riveting things— right now in California we have ICU staffing ratios of max one RN to two patients.

These are going to go out the window any minute now, alas (although I understand why, see above) but that's optimal conditions. Why? Because it's safer and produces better patient outcomes. Markedly. You can look up the literature on your own.)

What gets you your own nurse, depending on the facility?

ALL THE THINGS THAT HAPPEN WHEN YOU HAVE COVID.

Are your lungs shot? Do you need to be turned on your stomach to maintain lung function? Do you need to be medically/chemically paralyzed to keep you on your stomach for your lung function? You might be a 1:1!

Do you require multiple pressors—blood pressure medications that can require frequent titrations—to keep your blood perfusing to your organs so they keep working? You might be a 1:1!

Did covid fuck over your kidneys? Do you require continual renal dialysis? Note: not the kind your elderly relative gets MWF—we're talking live-time 24/7, right at the bedside, plugged in and don't stop washing your blood, dialysis. If so, you might be a 1:1!

Are you getting ECMO? This is the heart-lung machine you hear people talk about on TV—where all of your blood is being siphoned into an external device that both pumps and oxygenates it for you so that your heart and lungs can recoup. You might be a 1:1!

Did covid give you clotting issues that gave you stroke-like symptoms that require frequent neuro checks, so we know that you're not getting worse and/or requiring surgical intervention? Or are you experiencing numbness and tingling in your legs from showering clots due to covid? You probably aren't a 1:1, but you maybe should be!

ARE ANY OF TWO OF THE ABOVE THINGS HAPPENING TO YOU?

Three?!?!

YOU SHOULD DEFINITELY HAVE YOUR OWN NURSE SO YOU DON'T DIE OF COVID.

(Also? If any of the above things sound scary/interesting, as they should, please Google them and you'll see why not just anyone can magically pop up to my floor and function.)

G) OTHER REASONS we can't take people off the streets to be ICU nurses:

We have access to a lot, and I MEAN A LOT of narcotics.

We're also in isolation gear all the time with covid. Getting into isolation gear mode—it's a state of mind, and a nursely way of being.

You remember that completely embarrassing video of FL Gov. DeSantis wearing his mask wrong?

How about being in a room where if you did that, you might die?

Or those gross super-spreader shots of, who was it, Bill Barr? Sneezing, wiping his nose, and shaking hands with people at that confirmation party in DC?

I don't want to work with people whom that shit hasn't clicked for—which, if you look at how many people are still fighting masks IS A LOT OF PEOPLE—and honestly, it's not ethical to work with them, either.

I don't want to take some newbie and have them get covid because they're not as hyperaware as I and my fellow nurses are, covid they'll then take home.

Some people aren't born paranoid.

Those people shouldn't become ICU RNs.

G) SOME LAST THOUGHTS:

So Cassie, you ask, if you can't take people off the streets and turn them into ICU RNs, who can you cannibalize from the rest of the hospital?

Whelp, part of the problem right now is that covid's all over the hospital. They're using ICU capacity as the official metric because we see the sickest of the sick—there's no place to go from us but home, heaven, or hell—but honestly, looking at the board: all floors of the hospital are getting evenly hit. It doesn't do us any good to snag a med-surg nurse or a stepdown nurse (the next level down from ICU, internally), when those floors are hurting just as bad as we are.

I know Newsom wants to crash course ICU RNs. I haven't heard any more from that since Stanford said "eff you," but....

Have you ever started a new job and wondered where the fuck the copier was? And then once you found it, why the fuck it required a keyed-in password or a badge, because, like, what, they can't afford copy paper or some shit and want to make sure you're not making posters for your lost cat?

Hospitals also have workflow.

I'm not saying they're impossibly complex. But I am saying that it's one thing when you can't find the secretary to tell you how to use the copier, and IT IS AN ENTIRELY DIFFERENT FUCKING THING IF YOU DON'T KNOW HOW TO FIND THE CRASH CART.

Like, all hospitals have the same shit inside them. But they're not built the same, organized the same, stocked the same, etc., past all the science shit.

Nurses with prior nursing experience who come to the ICU get 6 months of ICU-specific training.

Traveler nurses with ICU background still get a few days' orientation.

And what they both get, in Normal Times, perhaps most importantly, is plenty of staff around them that they can ask for help.

If your staff is new, or less experienced, or trapped inside an isolation room doing continual dialysis/ECMO all by their lonesome—there's just a brain drain. Sometimes the covid wing looks like a ghost town because we're all working very, very hard in our own rooms.

But usually? We ask each other for help/opinions/ideas ALL THE TIME. That's one of the most awesome things about being a nurse, is working with all my amazingly intelligent coworkers and being all, "Yo, I need back-up," and everyone figuring out what to do together. Someone will have seen something like what's happening to your patient now, only ten years ago, and remember exactly how to fix them. Some other coworker will remember that you have to hit that piece of equipment with four lbs. of pressure on the upper right-hand corner to make it behave. Some other *other* coworker will remember the oddly elaborate process that it takes to get sterile processing to send you a Dingle Hopper, which is the only component of the thing that you need to do immediately that you do not presently have.

(Please don't give me guff about non-optimal workflow if, again, you have ever had to badge into a copier in your place of business. Thank you.)

We're going into a dire time here, my friends.

I'll take those warm bodies that do that ICU crash course, no problem. [CA: California ended up not instituting this.] I'm not going to turn my nose up at people who know where shit is and have hustle.

But surely you can see, after I have wasted a PRECIOUS HOUR OF MY SLEEPING TIME TYPING ALL THIS, that between now and Jan 31st is going to be A BAD TIME TO BE HOSPITALIZED FOR ANYTHING.

NOT JUST COVID.

Because we're going to be short-staffed, we're going to be exhausted, we're going to be emotionally traumatized from being the LAST PEOPLE WHO WITNESS all the deaths that should've NEVER OCCURRED in the first place HAD OUR GOVERN-MENT ACTED LIKE A GOVERNMENT AND GIVEN A SHIT, we might have friends/relatives/coworkers out with covid—or lost people, personally!—and we're going to be sweating our asses off in n95 masks and plastic gowns, dehydrated and cranky, utterly unpretty and entirely irreplaceable.

H) SO, in closing....

We're gonna try and keep you alive, okay?

But like, please, meet us half-the-fuck-way?

Wear masks and don't go out if you don't absolutely have to. Don't troll Target for funsies. Don't go see your Grandma at Christmastime, I don't care how emotionally manipulative she is.

. . .

PLEASE FOR THE LOVE OF GOD AND SOME NURSE NAMED CASSIE—stay home.

I'm sure you're awesome and all, but I don't want to meet you in person.

And you sure as shit don't want to meet me.

– CASSIE

Rupert Murdoch gets vaccinated. (12/18/20)

12/18/20

I'm on break like a bitch while my new hire navigates her first covid comfort care.

I'm not always saintly, and some things you've just got to learn how to feel on your own.

We talked about what she was going to do before I left, and I gave her a shit-ton of morphine to administer.

12/18/20

For the afternoon crowd: the only reason we're not 100% full at my ICU right now is because my patient died. Lolsob.

12/18/20

They're starting to vaccinate here tomorrow. Transport and Emergency is going first.

Our temp boss just text blasted us all: "I promise I will let you know your times ASAP."

Subtext: please get off my junk.

12/19/20

I had a dream last night that Ted Cruz was signing death certificates at work with me.

We were in a big airplane hangar full of body bags going from table to table.

I got to shout at him as he walked away, so there was that.

12/19/20—password protected journal.

Going to get my shot on Monday!!!!

I know I need two vax for it to work all the way, but just BEING IN PROGRESS is such a morale booster, damn!

12/19/20

In depressing-news that-makes-sense alert: I hung out with an organ donor nurse last shift (being jealous that they don't see any covid action mostly, while they wanted to know what it was like) and: You can't donate organs if you've ever had covid.

12/20/20

16 hours till I get my vaccine, but who's counting?

Stanford's vaccine algorithm mysteriously puts members of administration and doctors working from home ahead of front-line emergency physicians. (12/21/20)

12/21/20

Gets vaccinated at 14:45. Offers to stay till 23:00. Yeeeeehawwww!

12/21/20

Shit is hitting the fan here. Wonder if I could stay till 3am and pull a 20-hr. shift.

Wonder if I did, would my husband kill me?

[CA: after this week we were officially told by management, no 20-hr. shifts.]

12/22/20

We have 11 nurses scheduled for Christmas and we're running 20 deep every shift right now. I'm reaaaaallly curious how that's going to go. Maybe they shouldn't have fired our manager?

—₊₊₊—

12/23/20—This series of tweets was written in response to Kirk Cameron holding a maskless carol singing service.

Lord please may covid get Kirk Cameron.

And I just may be in a bitchy mood, staring down the barrel of two 16-hr. shifts, tomorrow and on fucking Christmas, but I don't want him to get the gentle, "Oh, I feel warm" kinda covid.

I want him to be on a ventilator somewhere, considering his life choices.

Why does he think his Christmas is more important than mine? Than literally any other person out there's Christmas?

Why does his Jesus want him to kill people for his birthday?

How the fuck is it holy to go and convince your fellow men to put themselves in the line of fire?

What a perversion of everything Christlike and anything the actual Christ stood for.

I'm so fucking fed up with the Supply-Side Jesus that vast tracts of our government would have you believe in. The Jesus who only appears to worthy people who're already wealthy as they shove your chin into the mud with their boots on the back of your head.

Their version of Jesus, who requires that you risk your life for "the economy," like that's not a fucking joke. If an afterlife exists— something I no longer believe in, having been raised evangelical and then having had reality/nursing career burn all my faith out of me— but if, sweet if, there is an afterlife—I hope people like Kirk Cameron get to the pearly gates and God laughs at them, while everyone that they've endangered helps shove them into a hell where they are semi-conscious on a ventilator for all eternity.

12/23/20

I can't tell if this is post-book-finishing depression, everything-covid depression, pre-work depression, or just a natural sinking into myself to avoid all human contact until I've got to turn my brain and be "on" on for real tomorrow.

12/23/20—password protected journal

Got my vaccine on Monday!

Had today and yesterday off to recoup in case I had side effects (I did not!)

And now I've sold my soul to the hospital, prescheduling myself a ton. They're offering so much overtime, and we're so crushed and I'm so stupidly helpful. We'll see how everything goes. I've got back-to-back 16-hr. shifts tomorrow and Christmas.

I kind of shut down before big stressful events and I can feel myself doing that now. I was always the kid at the martial arts tournaments sleeping on their gear bag at the side of the ring between bouts. My shifter-animal is some kind of "very energy conserving hound" in between bursts of frantic activity.

I don't think I'll be writing at all for the month of Jan, with the way my work schedule's looking and if we continue to be as slammed as I think we are. There's literally no way we cannot be, alas.

I do have some plans for pleasure reading and for doing some very outstanding critiques for friends, so there's that to keep my brain running. And the third book in this side series will be waiting for me when I'm good and done with all this.

But right now I'm staring down the barrel of four 16-hr shifts a week for most of Jan. I just bought extra scrubs so I won't have to do as much laundry.

Just have to get through all this nonsense for a few weeks is all. If I pitch in strongly for a month I won't feel so bad about pulling back in Feb when it's my birthday.

I can do this. It starts tomorrow, let's goooooooooooooooooo.

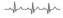

3379 deaths today, nationally, from covid, and 323,274 total, so far. (12/23/20)

—⎺⌄⎺⌄⎺—

12/24/20—ICU diary I did on twitter, part one:

0700: Get assignment, badge in. Discover temporary boss hasn't done our quarterly badge renewal, deal with help desk for 15 minutes while the nightshift RN slowly wants to die.

0715-0730: Get report. Two very sick covid patients (surprise, surprise), will call them A&B. Cross sign all hanging narcotics with outgoing RN.

0730-740: Plan my day. Call blood bank. Where's patient B's blood?

0745: Draw labs on A. Get a heating device on A; their temp is precipitously low.

0757: Ungown, drop off labs, hand phone to break relief nurse in case blood bank calls, go on break till 0825 and start typing this up, stay posted. (I haven't laid hands on patient B yet. They look good through the glass. But if I don't take my break, I won't get one.)

1100: I've been in a plastic isolation gown since I posted that last. I'm covered in sweat. Busy, busy. I'll go back later and fill y'all in. Out of gear right now and on the elevator to pick up remdesivir from the pharmacy.

Now at lunch break. In the past 4.5 hrs. I have:

Hung/replaced five IV bags

Given 20 pills

Given five-six liquid meds

Given six IV meds push

Given blood via a warmer, finished blood

Brushed both my patients' teeth

Cleaned their penises

Turned/repositioned two times/each

Drew more labs

Flipped my prone patient supine

Did an EKG

Talked w/MD re: heart rate/blood pressure/kidney function goals

Noticed/notified blood in my residual check of feeding tube

Got one patient's bowel program started

Notified MD that one patient is peeing way too much, indicative of possible kidney/neuro damage.

Talked 15 mins to one patient's elderly brother, listening and explaining compassionately without giving false hope.

Reported broken ceiling lift to engineering

Returned blood warmer to OR

Did all of the above safely for my patients; sake, coworkers sakes, ancillary staff's sake

1240: I haven't charted a thing yet, lololol.

1416: Just now out of rooms, again. Sitting down to chart. Cracking open my first Coke Zero.

1533: Done with charting and mostly caught up! Now to keep an eye on things—my patients are on seven blood pressure meds and five narcotic drips between them, plus one's paralyzed. All of these have different/optimal parameters that I'm steering them toward.

1538: Usually a patient on a paralytic is a 1:1 assignment here, because they're particularly vulnerable, but staffing is tight.

1545: My labs came back good, so no field trips to CT. A's temperature got fixed and most fires put out. Just have to wait to see when/if their lungs get better is all. 7.25 hrs to go.

1716: Helping out with breaks, getting everyone toward the finish line. Still copacetic.

1823: Finishing up all my end-of-shift tasks. Last labs, turns, emptying foleys, making sure my lines are labeled, etc. I'm going to be break relief on nights from 7pm - 11p. I'll make sure everyone gets a break here on the covid side, taking care of 10-plus patients in quick succession.

1826: There's no one coming in to replace me at 11p yet, so the break I give them may be the only one they get. I still have one Coke Zero left in the fridge. This is good, actually: It'll keep me awake having different patients, and I know most of these patients. They've been here 4 weeks.

1915: Gave report to incoming RN, got report from outgoing break relief, did count of narcotics drawer. Taking my own short break before diving into everyone else's. Reading LJ Shen's new book *The Villain*. Merry Christmas to me.

2034: Just watched a patient who has been here 28 days. Possible intubation coming down the hall, high-flow oxygen is no longer cutting it. Helped an RN make another patient prone for lung function. Waiting for RT to come help change an endotracheal (breathing tube) holder on another patient, already prone.

2056: They took our rapid response RN (the ICU nurse who goes to emergencies where a lower-level patient's about to be escalated) for an admit on the other side. By some miracle, high flow patient's oxygenation has gotten better. Maybe they won't get intubated tonight.

2100: Our 20-year-old patient who is self-proning has called to ask for permission to unprone to pee. He is very interested in living. I like that in a patient.

2200: Looking like charge is going to get pulled for care tonight. Desperately trying to get last two nurses out for their breaks here now. Won't be any more breaks past 11 when I leave. Unlikely to have any break relief tomorrow at all.

2300: I've got two nurses out, racing the clock. They'll be back at 2330 and then I go home. These were wraparound breaks, their second breaks taken very early while I'm here. I *may* have been out of ratio compliance for the past two hours. (Theoretically, of course.)

2327: Badged out! Speedwalking to my car. Home, shower, 5mg Ambien, and it all starts again tomorrow.

12/25/20

If you hear someone saying, "my friend who works in the

ICU says things aren't so bad" right now, ask them about their Canadian girlfriend.

12/25/20—ICU diary I did on twitter, part two:

Those who are about to try to save your lives on Christmas salute you.

My favorite RT called this morning and said coffee was mandatory, so I drove a little further out and got our orders. I have the same pair of patients from yesterday.

One of my coworkers has only had three days off in Dec. Another stayed here till 11 last night with me, doing a 16, went home, napped, and came back at 3 am.

Got this from Staffing this morning. (Note, they did not "try everything," seeing as today's staffing has been dire for weeks and they just started to give a shit yesterday.) My coworker who worked 16 yesterday and who came in at 3 a.m. today is now in charge and break relief.

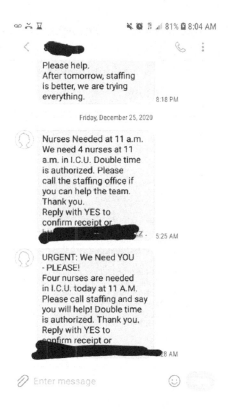

I'M ADDING these asides not to make you feel bad for us, but just so that you realize how dispensable we are to administration. We get paid well, but we're expected to work like dogs in subpar conditions that will become blatantly unsafe in about three hours here....

Patient with low blood from yesterday got low again overnight. Blood warmer procured, waiting for blood bank. Cold patient yesterday now has a fever, alas. I get to coast some, though, because I know these patients and their flow, which is good.

One of my co-workers worked 21 hours in a row this past week. You may remember Monday, when they would have been eager for me to stay for 20. Administration says now that's illegal, don't. But if they send four night-shift nurses staying over home at 11....

0911: Patient on high flow last night that I thought was going to get intubated just did.

1056: Makes "upcoming shark sound from Jaws." They've got five mins left to find three RNs.

1131: Freshly intubated patient now getting chemically paralyzed to maintain lung function.

1242: So busy. So tired. I got to eat some though.

1244: Lo-fucking-l

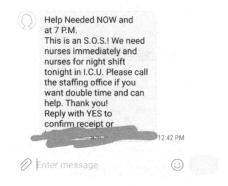

I FORGOT to thread this thought, but seriously, it feels like I'm dating the staffing office and I'm ALREADY HERE.

Night shift RNs came in early and saved us. Have enough staff to flip my manually proned patient back over now. [CA: we do this to check on people's lung function and hopefully, if they're doing better, they can withstand breathing on their backs for longer and longer periods of time until they're "normal" again.]

1816: ALMOST DONE WITH DAYSHIFT and then to be break relief on nights. I'm going to need this third Coke Zero injected into my soul.

2008: This Coke Zero is like drinking water. Two nurses on break, "theoretically" watching three patients, trying to get everyone through.

2010: You can tell how tired I am by how little I've cursed on here today. I'm titrating this Coke Zero like my life depends on it.

2303: Oh God, they found coverage. I can go home slightly early.

I was totally going to take off my surgical mask to eat this massive piece of peppermint bark I stole on the way out to my car, but I thought, no let's just hold off, and around the corner of the building ran into a big group of people, all in masks and looking under the weather, heading in.

12/26/20

Today's been a flat day. *Looks at care tag, reads instructions*
I've got to try to exercise and get outside some tomorrow.

12/27/20

You know it's bad when they take you for fractions of a shift. I'm not going in personally, don't worry, just bracing to do another 16 tomorrow.

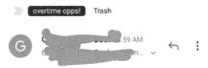

Re: HELP - DAYS TODAY 12/27

overtime opps! Trash

Desperately looking for help today. We are short 2 nurses at 11am and 3 nurses at 3pm! Double time is still on the table as well as the appreciation and gratitude of your coworkers! Come in for whatever works for you - 3, 4, 5, 6 etc. hours. Nights - come on in early if you like also?

Thanks

12/27/20

I fuckin' hate this guy so much. I really wish it was him gargling for life at the end of a breathing tube than literally anyone else I've had to take care of for the past nine fucking "GOP GONNA DO NOTHING ABOUT COVID" months.

[CA: This was in response to Marco Rubio saying dumb shit. Politically astute readers will note I don't even need to share what dumb shit it is that Rubio said here, because they know all of his "Let me post a Bible verse to Twitter like I care about saving human lives, even though I clearly don't" shit is dumb.]

12/27/20

I could've given birth to a child in the time I've been taking care of covid patients, and then that self-same imaginary baby, nearly 14 days old now, would've been more useful to me taking care of covid patients THAN LITERALLY ANYTHING THE GOP HAS DONE DURING THAT SAME TIME.

That baby might've helped repopulate the NEARLY 350,000 PEOPLE WHO'VE DIED ON THE GOP'S WATCH WHILE THEY STOOD AROUND WITH THEIR DICKS IN THEIR HANDS—EVEN THOUGH NOW THEY ALL HAVE THEIR ARMS OUT FOR SHOTS.

12/27/20

My elderly parents, who I, even as an ICU RN, could not talk out of making a cross-country move and visiting all of their relatives along the way, are in Texas now. My aunt and uncle, who they saw in AZ, are now covid positive and my mom is sick.

I just want to throw up and cry.

If my mom does have covid, which seems likely, seeing as my parents visited my aunt/uncle two days prior to their positive diagnosis—they hung out with my brother's wife's whole family on Christmas, including her elderly parents as well.

I try and I try and I do nothing but try and for what? What is even the point of all this trying? I am breaking myself, and for why or who or who the fuck cares?

All I want is for people to listen to me and do the right thing. That's all I've ever wanted. I don't know why it's so hard when it could've been so easy. I'm going to go cry with my husband now.

I'm lost.

12/27/2020—password protected journal

All you beloved fuckers better stay home because I need someone to actually listen to me.

All of this can't be for nothing. I can't take it anymore if it is.

12/28/20

My mom does have covid.

I'm explaining to her how to prone herself. Texting my dad with quarantine instructions for himself and everyone in my brother's household and everyone they saw over Christmas.

While at work.

Taking care of covid patients.

For my current patient, I asked our MD what the plan is, and he was all, "find more people to carry the coffin"—by which he means involve a few more services, so we can get this family to understand that the patient won't make it.

My husband asked if I should come home. I can't. Can't change anything for my mom; she's three states away. Can't bone over my coworkers. My patient is a 1:1, and we're going be short at 11 as is. Told him my plan was just to be a mess on Twitter, so here we are.

Brace yourselves.

Holding it together okay so far. Work is good busy. Shoving feelings into feeling hole. Went to talk to my coworker whose dad bought a gun pre-election, worried about the "antifa" and we had a good I FUCKING HATE FOX NEWS moment together.

Remembering when my parents told me, "we're killing the economy," and "God knows when it's your time," and I want to fucking fire hose that shit like a dragon now. I pushed back on it at the time, to no effect. So angry still. More angry than anything else.

Basically, doing what they were doing when they were doing it made this inevitable.

Except for the part where it didn't have to happen at all.

Made an appt for my psych-medication MD on my break.

Man, it's a really good thing I got my first vax shot. If I hadn't, my mood, already wafer thin, would be subterranean.

Work wants me to stay for a 16. I laughed pretty hard and said no.

Almost didn't switch my masks before I went into my patient's room. My game is not tight today. Thinking about calling in sick tomorrow.

I'm going to go ahead and go in tomorrow. I might need to spend that sick day later in the months on edits for this book [CA: the fiction book I was working on at the time] and I'll keep my easy assignment.

My patient's going to die no matter what I do, so the cold calculus of the covid nurse is on full display here.

Sorry, it ain't pretty. If they had a chance, I'd care more, but since they don't, barring a time machine and going back to pre-Thanksgiving, it is what it is.

You've got to wrap your heart in spikes to do this job.

12/29/20

Got my second vaccine appointment on the books!

12/30/20

I've gotten a lot of new followers lately, and I worry that you new people think I'm actually a responsible adult, so I wanted to say some ground-rules:

1) I'm not a hero (as per my pinned tweet) nor am I actually nice. I am good, but I'm not nice. There's a difference.

2) I no longer have an inside voice.

3) I curse. A lot. And shout. A lot. I am angry. A lot.

4) I don't want your sympathy for me personally most times. I'll let you know when I do. For my patients, yes, but not for me.

5) It weirds me out when people are too nice to me. I don't have a framework for accepting kindness. I also don't need

much of it, honestly. If I thrived on anything but exhaustion and spite I wouldn't be working in the ICU, even before all this happened.

6) People want to know what they can do for me, and I get that—it's human—and I appreciate intellectually that you want to bond. And I say things that sound bad sometimes and you might get worried. But that's now-me. Tomorrow-me likely won't even care.

7) For instance, I've got blisters on my fingers from bagging my patient for so long yesterday, which is quite fucked up. But in the story I'll tell about this in the future, if I even bother to (because it's one drop in a vastly shitty bucket), I'll probably laugh it off. [CA: She would not laugh it off. In fact, this one moment would fuck her up for quite some time. Also, I recognize now that telling traumatic stories and laughing is a fucked-up thing to do, but sometimes you do it because you have no other context for those stories. If you don't laugh, you'll cry, and if you start crying, will you ever stop?]

8) I have (thrillingly self-diagnosed) PTSD. But so does every healthcare worker currently in America, so I neither feel special, nor will I want special treatment for it later. [CA: More lies.]

9) I just like to write things out. Very much always have. Very much always will. I wouldn't remember anything otherwise. I know I can seem emotional in the moment and I ride that to function, but it's OK, I do all right.

10) So that's why I tweet. I am not looking for attention. I view this as kind of a weirdly intermittent blog where other people can interact. If it makes you happy to interact with me, you are welcome to do so. I may not have bandwidth for more than a "like" back, though. Sorry.

11) Being ever so slightly more popular now gives me the heebies because I don't want to let anyone down, but at the

same time I need to hoard my own resources for me, at the moment. That said, I'll answer any medical questions you've got at the drop of a hat. DM at will.

12) In summation, I'm OK; hopefully you're OK; we're probably not going to be besties because I have no room at the inn, but if you want to stick around for the ride I'm A-OK with that, as long as you don't make demands on me socially.

You need a nurse though, and I'll come running.

Pharmacist in Wisconsin intentionally destroys 500 doses of vaccine. (12/30/20)
[CA: He was just sentenced to three years in prison for this, in June 2021, and rightfully fucking so.]

12/31/20—Two Nurses Talking newsletter

DON'T GO OUT

Please.

Just don't.

I'm putting this placeholder post in here now, and we'll see if I get a chance to change it between now and the 31st.

I have every intention of coming back here and writing something moving and thrilling that makes you totally reconceptualize your viewpoint and gives you the munition you need to explain to everyone else in your life why you're staying home as much as possible, and not only that but something SO MAGICAL it CONVINCES THEM TOO to stay home, like some "I clap for fairies!" fever dream that flows outwards from all of our well-meaning hearts to somehow inspire and heal our nation and get everyone who is currently a dickwad to stay home and not breathe on anyone else in the new year.

I want to water your crops and help you regrow your field of fucks that has so long been barren. I want to make your skin glow, I want your tiktoks to go viral, I want you to feel whole and well and loved.

Barring my abilities to make any of those things happen though, the only thing I can control or give to you is this:

If you're making sacrifices right now, you're not alone, and your efforts haven't been forgotten.

I appreciate you. Thank you for believing in me and what I'm telling you from the hospital. Thank you from the bottom of my heart for not making my job harder.

This year has to get easier. It just has to. For all of us.

We just have to make it long enough to see it, is all.

We can do it.

For the rest of the world, I don't care about them, and I don't trust their motives.

But if you signed up to read this, you signed up for a reason, because you cared about learning, and your health, and my health, and others.

We're going to get through this and we're going to get out on the other side, together.

<3
Cassie

12/31/20

MD walks by: Hey, what was that patient's baseline?

Me: Well, 6 people were holding him down in ED before they paralyzed him.

MD: So purposely moving all extremities then?

Me: Uh... yeah? I guess?

MD: Have you seen him move?

Me: I have him lashed to the bed like Odysseus.

12/31/20

This year was trash in so many ways, but I had a really lovely support network, including some of y'all, and everyone here nicely tolerated all the times I was losing my shit and looked/felt/was crazy. Thanks for that.

Also I wrote four books, which is AMAZEBALLS, and my garden is now the shit (largely because of my on-Ambien spending habits), and ALL OF MY REAL-LIFE FRIENDS have taken covid seriously! Which really means so, so much to me.

This year has tried my soul and conscience in so many ways, but I've spoken my truth and done my best and that's really all I can ask of myself.

I'm not perfect and I'm going to screw up some, but as long as I'm smart enough to ask for help and/or the right questions, it's all going be okay. Especially after my second shot.

In summation, most of you RL friends already know how I feel about you. I love you, that's just how it is, and I'm really glad you're still around.

All you other people that my phone has made up for me seem pretty rad too, so keep on keeping on.

And we'll get through this dumb shit together because fuck if I'm letting the bastards win.

See you guys next year.

JANUARY 2021

1/1/21

Let's kick off today.

Another 11 in the saddle or 15 if you're nasty.

Too early for a Janet Jackson joke? Never. There might be more free association than usual here today, though.

Respiratory, re: my patient: Why are his hands like that?

Me: blood, dirt, and homelessness

Took a short nap on break. It was a good call. Gave my coffee time to work. Luckily my patients are chill.

I'm pretty tired, but so is everyone else? So we're all granting each other quite a bit of grace today.

Oh wait, I knew I had a depressing story. A coworker interrupted me last tweet and I got derailed. Anyhow, literally everyone that's left their house unsafely has covid now. We got a suicide in yesterday. They had covid. (These facts are unrelated, except that covid is everywhere.)

There's an NP who flies back and forth from their southern home state who wasn't 100% on the mask train this summer and right now I have a barely controllable, and rationally irrational, amount of rage at them. Got to simmer down.

I talked with a coworker a long time yesterday about how, from here on out, we're going to be disgusted with vast swaths of humanity, and yes.
    100%.
    How can I look someone in the eye in the future, knowing that they didn't wear a mask?
    I mean just like you shouldn't fuck Republicans, you also shouldn't fuck anyone who thought it was okay not to wear a mask.

Locked in for the 16. 12 hrs. left. That'll be 104 hrs. of work this paycheck. If you do the doubletime math, it'll be like I worked 136 hrs., paycheck wise, with all my overtime and two holidays.

This is also why I feel weird with people getting me stuff right now Things suck, but at least out here in CA, I'm well compensated.

Muttering "you're tough, you can do this" to myself under my napping blanket on the couch in the waiting room, only to discover four other people quietly breaking in there when said blanket is removed. At least they agree I'm tough, though?

Coworker: Are you back tomorrow? Me: Fuck no.

Might not have to pull a 16. They're trying to pull a new hire off of orientation. I'm feeling slightly more alive, thanks to Coke Zero.

Psych. They need me till 11. I shouldn't have gotten my hopes up.

I just got to do a massive wet-to-dry dressing with a coworker though—and the vending machine gave me an extra KitKat—so today's looking up!

Punch-drunk tired. Luckily same patients. On autopilot.

One hour to go. Just ate a Snickers and my extra KitKat.

Walking out to my car! I want to sleep more than I want another 15 minutes of double time.

There is a line of cars with headlights on out here. And quite the line heading into the emergency department

Home! Thank God! I didn't want to let on how scared I've been for the past four hours that they were going to transfer out one of my easy patients and give me a shitty admit.

Bullet dodged. Bedtime!

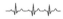

1/2/31

Me: Finishes, polishes 6000-word deeply personal non-fic essay and gets it ready to show the world.

Also me, three hours later, to my paranormal-romance fiction coauthor: Look, all I currently know about these characters is that I am 100% positive they need to have anal sex.

1/3/21

I really don't want to go to work tomorrow. What I want is a week off and a hot tub and to stare at the sky thinking about book stuff, plus-minus being high.

1/3/21

Lying in bed, realizing that my New Year's ambition is, as it has almost always been, to take less shit and to have an even shorter fuse when it comes to dealing with intentional ignorance.

1/4/21

Only working a 12 today, no matter what.
   I got excited that I was on the non-covid-19 side again, then found out I have the covid overflow patients over there.
   I think it's impossible to overstate how little I want to be here today. I have tomorrow off, though.

My mask denier (don't fucking ask, I know) coworker is on break with me now.
   Good thing I already ate. Putting my mask back on.

1/4/21—Two Nurses Talking newsletter

Covid, Fox News, America, and me

This is going to be long; bear with me and settle in.

As a lifelong nerd with a writer's morbid side-interest in all the ways people can die and a habit of following all sorts of people on Twitter, I saw Italian ICU videos of nurses caring for coronavirus patients back in March. [CA: that I mentioned prior] I knew then that covid was going to be bad, and emailed my parents as much, asking them to stay home and be safe.

At the time, they told me they would.

But they were lying.

I CHOOSE to believe that they didn't always mean to lie.

I think early on, in early spring, when it looked like this was controllable and it was spreading slowly (except for poor NYC), everyone, including them, had Really Good Intentions about pitching in and stopping this thing in its tracks.

But then politics got involved and fucked us all over.

MY PARENTS, like many of your parents, perhaps (many people over 60, according to the ratings metrics) watch Fox News. And all of a sudden it became a red state/blue state thing, where the red states said "fuck y'all" and hoped we'd drown, because apparently being up on germ theory is not a requirement for public office.

My parents visited in late spring.

This was after the Easter fiasco, where my hospital had the biggest surge (at the time) of covid patients in our hospital system. When I didn't have enough gowns for a whole shift. When our bosses were marking out little dotted lines with tape on the floor inside covid patient rooms, saying that we could go safely so far into the room—but not a millimeter further!—safely, without gear on, to conserve gear. When we were begging n95s from the community, from people's wildfire stashes and from professional painters.

So there we were in my backyard, hanging out, and my parents start telling me things about "the economy" and "God knows when it's your time."

I'm staring at them, feeling dumbfounded.

Here I am, telling them I'm drowning—literally drowning. My job has never been more frightening or worse—and I'm a fucking tough lady. I was a burn nurse for a decade and I'm covered in 60-plus hours of tattoos—and they're all parroting Fox News talking points at me.

I'm watching people die of something that we don't know very much about, whose transmission capabilities we were (at the time) still not 100% sure of. I'm watching videos of nurses in China in fucking bunny suits while I'm being given sneeze guards and being told it's important for me, the person in the literal line of fire here, to worry about the economy?

Because the stock market is more important than the human lives I'm attempting to save?

Including my goddamned own?

My choices are to either call them out on their bullshit or to sit there dumbfounded, as my soul sinks like an anchor into the molten core of the earth.

I sit there. We've had these fights before. Been having them ever since Trump got elected. I know I'm not changing their mind, so why try? I'm so good at fighting for my patients, but I'm really, deeply lousy at fighting for myself.

My mom emails me later to tell me that I "seemed depressed."

I email her back to say, "Actually, I'm suicidal," because it's true, and I block her for a bit for my own mental health.

· · ·

SOMETIME IN THE summer my brother watches Pland*mic. (I put the * in there because I don't want it to be searchable—I don't want a flock of conspiracy weirdos showing up here and debating me over an easily discredited and entirely bogus video about absolute bullshit.)

He texts me, "They pulled it from YouTube. They must be scared of it being true!"

I text him back, "YouTube pulled the video of me calling him the best brother ever. It must be true!"

He sends back a laughing emoji.

After that, he sends me a few "people who wear masks are lemmings" memes—and I know we're both leaning hard into my mother because eventually she snaps and emails us both that: "Everyone has opinions about covid."

Well, just as one does not simply walk into Mordor—no.

One does not simply 'have opinions' about covid.

There is science. And there are facts. And what's true is true and what's true is right.

IMMEDIATELY AFTER DONALD TRUMP got elected, I began to worry about the consequences of living in a post-truth society. Right around the same weekend a(nother) Black man was shot in the back, while running away, on video, and the cop who shot him got off scot free—just as that one guy took his gun into the pizza parlor to search for the democratic pedophiles his despicable corner of the internet had told him were there.

I happened to be up at my parent's house that weekend and tried to use those examples to explain things.

We were literally watching a man get shot in the back. Running away. Not to get a gun—just running away from a cop.

And the cop got off.

And then that other damn fool read enough stupid shit about codewords that he believed his Pizzag*ate stuff, and couldn't be bothered to use his own brain to think things through.

He was so sure he was going to get to be the hero. (We'll come back to this, I think.)

I knew then that the writing was on the wall.

I just had no idea that it would ever get this bad.

I HAVE a friend who watches the political ball as intensely as I do—sometimes when things get hot, we'll email each other several times a day. (Hi Dave, lol.)

And he said something wise to me awhile back, and it was this: "You know, your parents have been on the receiving end of weapons-grade psy-ops for years now, right?"

And I think about that a lot. Sometimes it's the only thing that allows me to approach this situation with any equanimity.

My own mother once told me that protestors were paid, knowing that I was flying my dang self out on a SPIRIT AIRLINES REDEYE to go to the first Women's March four years ago. I told her that that's what they want you to think, so that it dehumanizes people when they get hit by rubber bullets.

No progress was made on either side.

Fuckin' Fox.

I REMEMBER when Trump got elected, how devastating that was.

And I'll be honest, my first (of many) dark thoughts when covid hit was—shit, this is going to be what bones us.

You see, up until then, yeah, the GOP had been being maliciously incompetent, but I thought surely—surely—this will be the moment that they set all that aside. They'll get the government together enough to function and "fight" covid, for some degree of fighting, and then Trump'll spend the next eight months patting himself on the back for doing a better job than some other country.

And the people who trust Fox news in this country will believe that he saved us, that he did a good enough job, that there Was No

Other Way, and because he's white and he has a dick, and, for an oddly masochistic segment of the population, because he is a dick, he'll get voted in again.

I knew the evil ran deep—I'm not blind, and I've been fighting against it ever since his election—but up until then I had just assumed the evil was some sort of generic uncaring thing, or at the most, specifically perpetrated on other ethnicities. Note: I'm not saying this is okay; I'm saying it's what I thought it was.

But of course they'd figure out that even white people travel. That we all move from state to state, in cars and on planes, that we all go to churches and malls and grocery stores and breathe the same air.

They'd realize—*wouldn't they?*—that ignoring the biggest public health crisis of our entire generation would murder hundreds of thousands of people, and they'd do something about it.

Right?

SOMETIMES I SIT AROUND and wonder who first thought it was okay to say that it was okay for some other segment of the population to die.

Like, who was the Chuck Yeager of that shit, that someone from Sinclair Media group sent them a memo which was all, "Yeah, it's okay if grandma goes, whatev's—just be sure to sell it on the air," and to which they were all, "Sure. Absolutely. Six o'clock."

You might be tempted to grant them some grace, and say, "Hey, they were in an at-will work state, trying to keep their job, and they needed the health insurance," to which I would say, "Yeah, like the Nazis needed bootlickers," but I digress.

The point is, someone, somewhere, thought that it was acceptable to start ticking off human lives as though deaths were inevitable and things that caused or hastened those deaths were necessary. [CA: now that I'm doing this project, I realize it was Larry Kudlow. Eff you, Larry.]

. . .

FAST FORWARD TO the middle of October. Our case load has lightened significantly, my brain's doing better—God bless the Bay Area, people taking shit seriously, wearing masks all over, I'm so proud of all of us—and I feel safe driving up to my folks' place to hang out, outside of course, in my n95.

We all go on a walk, and my mom tells me she wants to move.

record scratch

I'm conflicted. I realize, yeah, it's probably better for them to move away from me, their thorny-yelly-judgy-daughter, from their POV. I'm angry that I've lost the past seven months of hanging out in person with them because of covid. And I'm also angry at Trump for having fundamentally changed the nature of my relationship with them, although I know that he and Fox likely only exploited what was already there.

So I'm okay with them going out to Texas, to be with my brother, amongst more like-minded people. If you love someone, set them free and all that.

But—not-the-fuck-during-a-pandemic.

THUS BEGINS my second phase of efforts at keeping them safe.

Because there's no financial reason for them to be in a rush. Texas, as everyone knows, even in Oct/early Nov, is becoming a hotbed for covid. I tell them they should wait for Spring, till everyone gets vaccinated, people will still want houses and be thrilled to spend money, etc., etc., etc.

I know I've been "the emotional" one in the past. So I send them emails dry as mummies, with screenshots regarding Dallas ICU capacities. I preface everything with, "I hope you know I'm only telling you these things because I love you," even as I explain germ theory to them like they're children. (Fuuuccckkk you, Fox news.)

I tell them that they only reason they've been safe so far is because Northern CA has been safe, and it has nothing to do with luck, their health, or them. It's just statistics, and stats can change.

Nope. Nothing I do or say matters. They're intent on moving. Two 70-plus-year-old people fly back and forth to Texas to stay with my brother, who has two kids, and I know they're all maskless indoors, right after Thanksgiving, to buy a house.

Sometime in the middle of all this I get sent a photo of them with six people over the age of 65 indoors, maskless, from different states, visiting them because they're moving—and my mom gets a head cold.

I try to convince her that means her mask game is weak (because it so does) but the movers (which I offer to buy her out from) are already booked, and that's that.

So in mid-December I go up there, to get a few personal possessions and to see them for the last time for quite some time—because I won't feel safe visiting them till they're vaccinated like me, or till my whole brother's family gets vaxed, because I know that even when my vaccinations finish (1/10, hallelujah) I could still be an asymptomatic carrier and as someone who has been doing her GODDAMNED BEST not to kill anyone else, I'm not about to fucking start now—and we have our final, local hang.

My husband asks me not to hug them. I lie to him and tell him that I won't.

Instead, I bring along one of the rain ponchos I had overnighted off of Amazon after work boned me on PPE that day—I bought a set of 20—just in case.

I don't actually wear it the day of though. I just park a block away from their house on my way home and pull off my top two layers of clothing and wipe all of my exposed skin with hand sanitizer and alcohol swipes before taking off my mask.

But driving home, I finally get it.

As a writer and as a nurse, I like to think I'm hugely empathetic and that I go out of my way to understand other people's POV.

Honestly, I was so sure of my rightness, that I hadn't ever tried to see from their POV, because I was so sure it was wrong.

And, yeah, they are wrong. Wrong wrongity wrong. Don't worry, this essay isn't going that way.

But I had my first glimpse into their recent lives.

They were going to restaurants. I haven't been to a restaurant since February. People from their church are visiting them with their kids to drop off cookies. My cousin's bringing over her four kids under twelve to sing Christmas carols to them, inside their house without masks on—I know because they showed me video.

I felt like fucking Ariel from the Little Mermaid on land for the first fucking time.

You mean I've been living this life of monk-like deprivation and extreme work conditions in an effort to maximize survival rates and... you... just... haven't?

No wonder they think I'm insane.

They have no context—absolutely none—for what I'm going through, as a nurse. Or what hundreds of thousands of people are going through, as patients.

And honestly, you, you reader at home, you might not, too.

So let me catch you up with a recent bon mot. I don't usually tell work stories this close to when they actually happened, but as this work story is happening in all sorts of ICUs right now, all over the country, I'm not really worried about anyone picking out any identifying characteristics.

We had an elder of a family at our hospital. They didn't want to have a family Thanksgiving, but another elder overruled them, and then someone from the younger generation got both elders sick, along with themselves.

Earlier this week I was taking care of the sickest of these three, and they were dying, and the only reason we allowed other family members in the room with me was because they'd all already had and survived covid.

I spent nearly two hours bagging this medically sedated, chemically paralyzed, on their stomach (just like in Italy) patient, because a ventilator alone couldn't provide enough pressure/force of air into their lungs to keep their oxygen saturations up so that they could stay "alive" long enough for everyone to get to say good-bye. I'm hyperinflating their lungs with an ambu bag so they semi-function, blowing their delicate feathery crevices out into the smooth inner surface of a balloon inside, trying to force the covid-ravaged tissue to accept air.

I sat there listening to them facetime in other family members who were praying for a miracle, saying that it was going to happen, when the simple answer was, the second I stopped bagging that patient, with the ambu bag between my legs like a thighmaster, pumping 30 times a minute, they were going to die.

WHILE I WAS SEEING my folks, I had largely resigned myself to their fate. They were going on a cross-country trip whether I liked it or not, but you know me, I can't not try. I knew they'd be driving across I-10 and be visiting other relatives all along the way. It seemed like the height of madness to me, you know? I knew they were going to get exposed. I just knew it.

And of course I'm their medical executor person, and they already know I have strong feelings about end-of-life care, so we talked about that. My stepdad used to be an LVN at an assisted care facility, and so we talk, again, and he says, "Not everyone needs to live. Not all life is life." (In his defense, I'm paraphrasing mightily for space.)

And—I agree with that sentiment. Working where I do, I see a lot of people kept on far, far past their time, in my opinion, although I realize that that is not a decision for me to make—because if I do, instead of the family, I'm on the slippery slope to eugenics—and it's the same line of thought that make a body count of 350,000 tolerable.

I point that out, and the conversation moves on.

THE DAY before I spend two hours of my life trying to give other people some sense of closure in theirs is when I find out that my mother has covid.

(You knew that that's where this was going, didn't you?)

She's better enough now that I feel safe talking about it, otherwise this would've been a vastly different essay.

I am shit at work for the rest of the day. I tell my coworkers. I tell the intensivist. Everyone is very nice. I want to go home. I want to cry, and throw up, and then cry again.

She caught it from my Aunt and Uncle, visiting them in Arizona. (FUCKING ARIZONA. WHO THE FUCK STOPS THERE IN A PANDEMIC? UNBELIVABLE.)

My mom tells me they seemed fine when they visited—my Uncle just got a tickle in his throat after they left. (I wonder why I've wasted my breath trying to explain asymptomatic spread THIS ENTIRE TIME.)

(And? Once more, with feeling, FUCK YOU FOX NEWS. You could've been using your platform for good, and keeping your predominantly elderly viewers alive with actual science, but no, SO FUCK YOURSELF.)

I'm on the fence about going into work the next day, truly. My mood is as flat as a very flat thing. And that's when shit gets scary. Everyone who's ever been suicidal before recognizes that. Suicidal people don't have manic waves of energy usually. They get very quiet and feel very thin. Like you could just slip out underneath an airlocked door.

But I know work's the solution for many of my moods—I do best when I'm focused on other things—and so I go in the next day, and that's when I get to be the nurse there with my patient.

Pumping their lungs with a bellows between my legs, buffered by my hands.

Listening to their entire family, present both in person and electronically, crying, praying, wishing that things could be different for them, as they make the kind of gut cries that come out from the center of your being. Like there's not enough air inside you, nor will there ever be.

Knowing that their bad decisions led to this particular outcome.

Knowing that shit like that's going on all over the nation.

Knowing that shit like this could very well happen to my mom.

I go on break when it's my time.

The way we're staffed right now, we're very lucky to get breaks. You either go, or you don't get them, and bagging someone's exhausting—I'm aiming for at least 30 times a minute on the monitor, 35/min was what the setting was on the vent and I'm not a machine —and remember I'm in isolation gear. N95 on, and in my plastic gown. I'm covered in sweat, like a high school wrestler trying to make weight running laps in a Hefty.

I go on break because I've seen this particular drama play out before, and I don't feel the need to be its lone observer. I find nothing Mutual of Ohama Wild Kingdom or Jacque Cousteau in watching other people's grief. I'm a sympathetic crier, so it's hard for me to witness it, harder still when I can't hug the people crying, and a thousand times harder when I can't stop doing what I'm doing because if I do my patient will straight-up die.

And by the time I get back, thirty minutes later, they're gone.

All of that effort, all of those tears, those hopes, those prayers, those strongest wishes and fervent desires—all that pain and trauma and likely emotional scarring—and all for what?

Nothing.

None of it had to happen.

Not one fucking drop.

At any point in time, the government could've intervened and created sensible proposals that saw everyone housed and fed for long enough to trace and end this thing.

At. Any. Point. In. Time.

Seventy million people—including some of my relatives—voted for a government which is actively trying to kill them.

I don't know what to do with that.

I can't bag them all, one by one.

Is it going to take one person in each of their families dying for this to stop? Like some sort of eleventh plague?

I honestly don't know.

Sometimes I look at the news and I give up hope.

EVERYONE I'VE MET ONLINE who is anti-mask or anti-vax views themselves as the hero of their own story.

They all think that they're the one person who really has access to What's Going On. That they're going to be the person to break the conspiracy open and prove that hundreds of thousands of health care workers and centuries of science are lies.

They believe themselves to be Lone Mavericks of the Truth, serving the God of Personal Freedom, like health-points can be earned on a video game system, where functional lung tissue is assured if you believe both in Jesus and that America is a meritocracy.

I can't entirely blame them, as a story writer myself.

I understand the allure of thinking that you're the one pointing the good shit out. I mean, look, here I am doing it, and playing devil's advocate. It's really satisfying to think you're right, no doubt.

But first, you've got to make sure you're right about the right things.

You've got to make sure you haven't been lied too. That you're not being manipulated. That Fox news isn't trying to get you to kill your grandmother because rich people think paying for her social security is a drag.

I KNOW we all want to be heroes.

That's why I became a writer. I wanted to be like the people who saved me, the authors of my youth.

And I'm telling you now, if you're not staying home as much as you can—and I really mean it, staying all the way home, getting groceries delivered if you can afford it, no trips to the salon, birthdays, restaurants, bars, pedicure—you're missing your chance.

Don't be the person who killed your friend/neighbor/grandpa.

Stop trying to play Conspiracy Hero, The Game, and start being a real one instead.

I'm sorry that wearing a mask doesn't seem majestic or involve diesel trucks or firearms—that they don't make movies out of people wearing scraps of fabric on their faces.

I'm sorry that we've spent so long making contrarianism a sport that both-sides-style news reporting makes seem legitimate, even as it leads people to their graves.

And I'm sorry that saying no to people who very much want to see you, and who are always going off to do fun things without you, makes your monk-like under-the-sea-life seem dull and bland in comparison.

But this—this right now, this very moment—this is actually your chance to be heroic as fuck.

If you stay home, I promise you, you're going to be like Superman, John McClane, and John Wick, all put together.

You'll be my hero.

Swear.

THE NEXT DAY I had blisters on my fingertips from bagging, because my fingernails were a bit too long.

It was the same day that my mom says she wishes I could fly out to Texas and help take care of her.

I tell her the truth—I wouldn't even fly out for her funeral, if she died. I tried to say it nicely though.

Because right now, today, I know I could very easily be an asymptomatic carrier—just like my aunt and uncle were, and like whoever killed my patient. I work with covid patients. I'm in and out of their rooms every day.

It wouldn't have been right for me to endanger a whole plane's worth of people for the trip, nor anyone on the far end when I landed. You can't keep an n95 on 24/7, you know?

If she were to have gotten sicker, all I could hope was that some other nurse would've taken care of her just like I would.

SO PLEASE BELIEVE me when I say I know this shit is hard. It's been downright fucking cruel and right now the government is tying itself into knots to not give you $2000 because it doesn't feel like you've earned it, like the last nine solid months of this shit haven't been enough. What the hell.

I can only hope Biden's administration does us better.

But until they can get there, we've got to save ourselves, okay?

And I know that's hard, too—like, I couldn't even stop my own mother from getting covid. (So what kind of nurse am I? Existential essays for another time, I suppose.)

I'm already scared of what will happen if Biden does his whole hundred-day mask mandate—will vast tracts of people rise up to fight him, like they did in Michigan, when that militia tried to kidnap their own governor?

But the alternative is to give up and say that this amount of death is okay.

Let me decisively, authoritatively, tell you—it's not.

There's no death from covid that's a good death. Or an easy death. They're all gasping for air as their lungs punk out and drown. Nobody talks about that, how torturous it is, if you're at all aware of things. That you will see your own death coming like the fucking shark from Jaws, until we intubate you, and then after that, well, a lot of times, good fucking luck. And if you survive that—rehab post-covid is definitely a whole other future essay.

HERE'S the thing they never show on those heroic stories we all grew up on—the aftermath.

Like, we all want to be the Heroes! Heroes! Heroes!

But they never show the afterwards in the story, where/when

after a certain small group of valiant people did the right thing just in time, when they return home no one believes them.

The heroes come back from blasting the asteroid away from Earth—and a subset of people say, "Nah, man, that asteroid never existed." Or they barely contain the alien invasion, and then people are all, "Aliens? What aliens? Fuck you!"

Maybe if we showed more of this happening in fiction, people would want to be heroes less.

Because I've been getting called a hero this whole goddamned time, and I can tell you, watching TV in my patients' rooms, listening to lies come out of loved ones mouths, and being a person of the internet—it feels like shit to me.

BUT—I don't actually want there to be fewer heroes in the world.

I just want people to be smart—to be heroes about the right thing.

To take stands that actually make a difference—to live lives that really matter.

Lying down inside a Costco like a toddler because they want you to wear a mask is in no way shape or form heroic.

You, Mr. Costco, who have been given the span of all of your days, with fine lungs to breathe and apparently whine with, and this is how you goddamned spend it?

Or You, Mr. Call People Pussies on the Internet for Wearing Masks and Think We're All Lying—or people tramping through Target for Instagram—don't you fools realize YOU ARE STILL ABOVE GROUND?!?!

And you could take such simple actions to keep others there with you?!?!

The bar for true heroism has NEVER BEEN LOWER.

You don't even have to go to war to be a hero right now, friend!

You just have to stay home and when you (very rarely!) go out— wear a mask.

That's... it.

It's so simple.

And if we'd all agreed just to try hard from the jump, if no one had tried to opportunistically pit us against one another, so many lives could've been saved.

(Fuck. You. Again. Fox. News.)

PEOPLE WHO KNOW ME ASK, "Well, have you talked to your folks about the irony of all this?" and the answer is, no, not yet, because I'm clearly more of a 6,000-word personal essay kind of woman.

The truth is, when people are sick (and my mom's still in the recovery phase) I try to keep my interactions with them therapeutic.

The runner-up truth is, that mentally, I can't afford to listen to any more lies.

Anywhere. From anyone.

If I hear one more lie, one more half-truth, one more "I'm staying home, except for this birthday party," one more "the economy," my head will explode.

PEOPLE ARE DYING WHO DIDN'T HAVE TO DIE.

BECAUSE OTHER PEOPLE ARE KILLING THEM.

BECAUSE FOX NEWS AND THE GOP IS FULL OF BULLSHIT.

SO HERE WE are at the end of this essay, and once again I don't have answers for you. I wish I did, but the situation on the ground is evolving (a phrase I'm sure I've heard in heroic movies in the past). I clearly don't know how to convince people that they need to stay safe, for their own sake and others'. I don't know how to fight the pervasive American exceptionalism that our current media feeds, that makes people think the solution is to pull apart instead of coming together.

I don't know what to do with a nation that thinks opinions are facts. Or that GoFundMes are an acceptable alternative to national-ized healthcare, for that matter.

I write to try to pull people's eyes off of the ground, to get them to look for the horizon.

I hope that when they do that, they can't help but also see their neighbor.

But all I really know is that I see you.

I want you to live, even if Fox news doesn't.

I think you deserve healthcare and safety and enough money to make staying home and safe financially worthwhile.

In fact, I think everyone deserves a chance to live. And none of us should be lied to about matters of public health along the way, seeing as your health really is everything.

It's pretty much all we've got.

Everything else in life is negotiable. But Health is literally Life.

Ask anyone about to drown.

So.

Writing this helped me. I hope reading it helped you. Maybe it made you a little angrier, or your heart a little softer, or you feel more firm in standing your ground in the face of Future Unmasked Events.

That's all I can really ask for, in the end. Small subtle changes. Repetitive ongoing acts of heroism. The strength to say, "I'm staying home, thanks," or to call out your crazy uncle on Facebook—or maybe just block him for your sanity's sake.

Just keep trying to go through life clean. Know that the decisions you make now may not seem big—but they are.

I'm sorry we can't fight aliens together to be the heroes of this story—in many ways, I'd rather be doing that than fighting invidious misinformation and propaganda from the government.

But we're only in the story that we've got.

– Cassie

PS: Buzz Aldrin once punched a Moon landing denier.

Now that's a hero.

1/4/21

One of my patients today "recovered" from covid a few months ago... but because of their lung damage they're still going to die.

1/4/21

Highlights of today include my RT spontaneously breaking into Mickey Avalon's "My Dick" in the elevator.

An entire ICU ward in Egypt runs out of oxygen and the event is caught on camera. (1/4/21)

Los Angeles County is running out of oxygen and has instructed ambulance crews not to bring in patients with a low chance of survival, so they won't occupy beds. The city of Atlanta reopens a field hospital to take overflow covid patients. (1/5/21)

1/8/21

So now that my own mother has covid (miserable but okay so far) after my Very Extreme Objections to her dangerous activities, and I've been so open about it at work, I've become all of my coworkers' "Why won't my parents just listen to me?" confessor, as theirs slowly get it too.

1/9/21

My mom, still recovering from covid, has pneumonia now and a UTI and I am three very far states away from her, wanting to puke.

Yeah, that was the wheels falling off, along with my last coordinated fuck.

Just sitting here outside in my garden, sobbing, worried about my mom. Going to go find my husband, take an Ativan, and cancel today.

1/10/21—I GOT MY SECOND PFIZER SHOT.

1/11/21

And for its next act [CA: after Twitter having banned Trump] I'd really, really, really like @jack to take anti-vax people off of Twitter. We could probably start with the people that think "your blood needs to be more alkaline" and work from there.

I'm being snarky, but I'm not kidding, anti-vax people are a clear and present danger to public health. Imagine if someone went around tweeting that you should take your batteries out of your smoke alarms all day. You'd realize they were a danger to themselves and others. Same difference.

We need to start playing hardball whack-a-mole with bad science takes until covid-19 is under control.

1/11/21

I can't tell whether this sense of impending doom is the lingering effects of 2020, being behind in edits, knowing we're short at work, my mom being sick, my brother sending me dipshit censorship memes re:Trump and Twitter, two days after 2nd-shot-itis, or just a general malaise.

I've got my brother blocked on everything but Instagram

because all I post there are succulents and he mostly posts his puppy, and he's still up in my grill with bullshit.

The temptation to message him back and be all, "how do you feel about Trump making mom sick?" is so high, but it's my fucking plant account.

1/12/21

Trying to decide if I'm "writing my truth" or just "showing my ass in this novel" again.

1/13/21

Long day on the covid side. Taking care of two patients who have, combined, been here for a total of 75 days. Both trached & pegged now. They're not going to make it; they're just circling the placement drain, with families in denial.

Two of my other long-term patients died over the weekend.

One was younger than me and seemed to be doing better before they utterly decompensated. We pulled up their last CT because the NP wanted to show me their lungs—scarred through and through.

The other, I talked to their spouse my last shift, after we turned them supine so the spouse could talk to their paralyzed form.

They were a family holidays death.

C'est la vie.

1/13/21

Management came by to see if anyone still needed to be vaccinated. They've got some Moderna they're going to have to toss if not, and we're all trying to get them to let us call our husbands like women trying to get their men on life rafts leaving the Titanic.

1/14/21

So a coworker drifted over, and we reminisced about the patients that died this past weekend, and then she was all, "is it bad that I don't feel bad anymore? I just...can't."

And then we had a big talk about PTSD and dissociation and what we're all just doing to get by.

1/14/21

I WANNA KNOW WHAT GOOD LUNGS LOOK LIKKKKKKKKKEEEEE. I WANT YOU TO SHOW MEEEEEEE.

1/14/21

God, 16 hrs. is so long. Are we fucking there yet?

Meanwhile my coworker from my PTSD chat earlier, still here with me because she is also a sucker, just walked by and said, "Yeah, no; not feeling things is fine," semi-sarcastically.

I'd hug her but we've got to wait another week.

Multiple states were led to believe there would be second doses of vaccines coming from a federal reserve created under the Trump administration. No such reserve exists. (1/15/21)

1/15/21

They opened up PACU for ICU patients again and had

to pull nurse educators to staff earlier so nightshift staying onto days could go home.

[CA: Nurse educators are still nurses, but they run all the skills day presentations, check certifications and what not. At my facility they are never expected to staff the floor.]

1/15/2021—password protected journal

Yesterday I had a patient and their family wanted me to put the iPad for the facetime like six inches from their face, so they could all shout at them for 90 minutes, trying to see if they would do something, or move, or anything, really.

They're all worried about the patient's brain (which is gone; they don't even have a cough or gag reflex) when their O_2 requirements are 70% (normal air is 21%) and their PEEP is 10 (normal lungs, five, max possible 16-20)—like even if they did miraculously wake up, after having been on heavy narcotics and paralyzed for the better part of a month, Their Lungs Are Still Trash And They're Not Gonna Get Better.

One of my coworkers walked by yesterday in the morning singing, "Another daaaaaay taking care of deaddddd peopllllleeee."

We're all feeling it. And by "it" I mean "the absolute futility of ongoing care in so many of these cases."

1/16/21

Low on RNs this morning, so they've taken all the orientees off of orientation and given them our "easy" patients, and me and another "strong nurse" have the hardest patients and are expected to help the ducklings along.

1/16/21

My husband, just now: Remember when we went on that cruise and sat with people we didn't know?

1/16/2021—password protected journal

I watched a bunch of news today at work and I've got to say, despite Depressing Political Things—Biden's vaccine team and plan looks amazing, and I feel like there's going to be a lot of follow through. He definitely is taking things seriously enough—and while it would've been nice to have competent leadership all along, better late than never!

1/17/2021—password protected journal

Talked to my mom today, who is now feeling much better, post-covid, even though it was the "sickest she'd ever been."

She was telling me how nice it was to be in Texas: it's so different, everyone goes out to restaurants and no one wears masks. She wanted me to visit sometime soon, and I was all, "Well, once it's safe," and then she told me she was worried about my/my husband's mental health from being such shut-ins and that....

I shouldn't "live in fear" about covid.

I told her I don't live in fear, I live in science, like I have been doing all this time, trying my hardest not to kill anyone else.

It was hard not to throw my phone across my backyard at that point, really.

Jesus wept.

Can't wait to go back to work tomorrow and take care of people who apparently did or did not fear covid an appropriate amount, thus ending their lives precipitously.

The US surpasses more fatalities from covid than there were in all of WWII. (1/17/21)

1/19/21

Somedays I wonder if this is how farm factory workers feel like.

I mean, they ostensibly have to keep the animals alive before they kill them, right?

Out of all the tweets I've thought about deleting this past year, this might be the one that I do.

1/20/21

Having an "I wish I'd taken a Flexeril last night" morning. It's too late to take one now.

Hopefully I can avoid being on any manual proning teams today.

1/25/21

The one-year-a-versery of dealing with all this shit coming up is fucking me up.

1/25/21—Two Nurses Talking newsletter

Hey there, it's Cassie again!

Thought I'd take a moment to go through and explain what "life support" really means, since it's a term that gets tossed around a lot but if you're not a medical person you might not have a great context for it.

At its broadest, life support is anything that you require to survive —makes sense, right? It's any therapy that, if you didn't have, you would die.

Before I get into the explanatory weeds here—sometimes we're taking care of people's grandmothers, who're writing them notes on facetime or sending texts, and they've got breathing tubes in or they're on three-four medications to keep their blood pressure up, and they are very much alive!

They seem very lively! After all, they're gesturing to you and writing notes!

But... they're still on life support. And if any one of those therapies were withdrawn, they wouldn't survive on their own, without it. It's kind of a hard disconnect sometimes.

So let's go system by system—I'll start with the lungs.

You might remember my big prior post on ventilators and ventilation, but basically, we put breathing tubes into people to help them survive.

Either they're currently not physically able to keep their airway open (and no airway means no air in lungs), or their lungs aren't functioning well enough to maintain their O_2 sats (oxygen is a requirement for life on the cellular level) so we need to take that function over for them.

As I've mentioned before in prior posts, you can only have a breathing tube in you for around two weeks, max. This is because, in general, the mere act of having a breathing tube in your mouth/throat —they're made with relatively hard plastic that can withstand bites— can cause mechanical erosion if left in too long.

No one gets sent home on a breathing tube.

Sometimes these can be downgraded to tracheostomies, those holes they can cut in your neck for breathing, and yes, sometimes people can go home with those—assuming you're still able to live at the settings that your home ventilation system can provide. But we don't send people home with trachs in that require too much pressure (the PEEP, the force with which we're pushing air into people), because if that PEEP can't be maintained, the patient would die.

Other mechanical objects that people can require to live include assorted CRRT machines—CRRT stands for continuous renal replacement therapy, and in general these people are very sick and also having breathing tubes and significant medication.

A CRRT machine is plugged into the patient via special lines into their veins/arteries and it siphons out blood, acting like a replacement kidney, processing out wastes and balancing electrolytes, before sending it back into the body.

You need your kidneys to survive, or something that can mimic kidney function periodically, like people getting dialysis. But what happens during normal dialysis is that you have fluctuations of fluid volume and can have swings in blood pressure. Some people are too sick to tolerate these, and some blood pressure medications can put more pressure on kidneys, so CRRT allows the dialysis to occur slowly, steadily, smoothly all day long. At my facility, and all the ones that I've ever heard of, people on CRRT machines are 1:1 RN assignments, because of the dangers of something going wrong with the machine or its attachment point to your body.

A lot of medications constitute life support—anytime you can't survive without something intravenously, it generically, kinda-sorta is.

This is where we get into the weeds a lot, when families call. They want to know what the vitals are, and sometimes some of them have some basic medical knowledge, so it's my job to explain things as I share.

Just because someone's blood pressure is 120/80 doesn't mean they're "getting better," if I'm maxed out on four different blood pressure medications, plus albumin, a solute-heavy fluid that attracts fluid intravascularly to increase blood pressure, plus frequent boluses of fluid.

Small nerdy aside: assorted blood pressure medications can: make your heart beat more quickly and more strongly, can increase pressure on your peripheral vasculature to bring circulating volume in, or can dilate your coronary arteries to promote out flow—there's a lot going on! And some drugs have more than one effect!

The numbers alone don't actually illustrate the effort going into keeping that patient alive—and people can't go home on four pressors, or even one, really. It's just not safe.

All of our "life support" mechanisms are just stop-gap measures to hopefully bridge assorted tissue functions until that tissue can heal, via infections clearing or surgical remedies performed.

But I think/feel like sometimes, especially now in Covid-Times (tm), when we talk to families, we tell them things in the abstract—yes, they've got a breathing tube in, etc., etc., etc., but we don't emphasize enough that that truly is life support.

More than once recently I've had family members on the phone upset by the frame shift of realizing their family member was on life support, and so I've started talking early and often about that, so that the gravity of the current situation is clear from the beginning.

By the time patients get to need ICU-level care, requiring "life support" is basically a given—in fact, on a normal floor you can't run any of these machines or titrate these medications like we do blood pressure meds.

It's not that people don't get off of life support—they do! All the time! Albeit less frequently in covid situations, alas—but I think knowing that that's how sick loved ones truly are gives people time to adjust. And if, sadly, things go poorly, then it doesn't seem to come out of left field.

It's hard out there for relatives right now. As thrilled as I am to not have visitors at the moment, because I like using their waiting room for my lunch break, it's really difficult for people who aren't at the hospital to understand all of what's going on, how busy we are in certain rooms, how many of us are in there and how often, and how much modern medical equipment is simultaneously running in the room, under our supervision.

I think sometimes that it's easier for people to believe "we did everything possible" when they're in there, seeing us do it, you know?

Because TVs and movies and people like Benny Hinn (to shout out a faith healer from back in the day) really lie about what life support entails, and that makes everyone's recovery look miraculous. Everyone's got some distant cousin's story, or they found some website on the internet—Lord, save us all from Dr. Google—that talks about an astounding recovery.

Families always say they're hoping/praying/waiting for a miracle, and what I kind-of want to say sometimes, but absolutely NEVER EVER WOULD because it wouldn't be therapeutic, is that a miracle is already occurring.

That miracle is this machine. Or this medication. Or me.

The miracle is happening, right now, this very moment. Your loved one would already be dead without our interventions happening here.

But we still might not be enough, and so for that, I'm ever so very sorry.

– Cassie

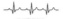

4077 people died of covid in America in one day. (1/27/21)

1/28/21

Sitting here waiting for my telepsych appointment to get refills on my prescriptions.

They're going to ask me how things are, and I have no way to even begin to contextualize that for them right now.

1/29/20—Two Nurses Talking

My last 12 hrs: how my most recent 1:1 shift went.

HEY PEEPS, Cassie again!

I just finished off a 12-hr. shift, although I'm waiting some time to push out this post, for HIPAA-adjacent reasons, and I thought I'd give y'all a summary of what went down while it's fresh in my mind.

First off, my patient was a 1:1 patient, which meant that I was their only RN, although I happened to have a new-hire/gopher that day, which was great.

The reason they were a 1:1 was because they were actively dying of covid.

Actively dying isn't a phrase you've probably heard before, unless you've worked with hospice. There are assorted stages to death, which I'm not going to get into here, but when I use the phrase I generally mean we've met the wall: there is nothing more that I, or even God, can do.

In theory, because this patient was dying, they could've given me another assignment alongside them, except for the fact that the patient was on ten different drips, and one of them was insulin. With a patient that busy, it would be cruel to give the bedside nurse another assignment, and it would've been inevitable that something would've dropped through the cracks, and then "actively dying" would've just become "plain ol' dead."

So, my patient had a breathing tube. We've talked about those before—what was ASTOUNDING this time was just how maxed this patient was. Their Fio_2 was 100%, which is never good, and their PEEP was *twenty-fucking-four*.

Just to illustrate how mad this is, I went around to all of my other coworkers, and I was all, "What's the highest PEEP you've ever seen?" And everyone said 22.

Like, 20 is what you start drowning victims off on. Normal is five!

24 is just asking for barotrauma—it's so much pressure I am literally surprised that this patient's lungs didn't just burst.

And then, they were vented to breathe at 32 times a minute. Sit around for a minute and breathe 32 times and see how that feels. It's probably double your normal rate.

All of this was in an effort to give their lungs as much O_2 as possible, percentage-wise, pressure-wise, and frequency-wise.

One of the reasons we had their breathing rate so high is because CO_2 (what you exhale from your lungs, what your body expires after taking in O_2 to make energy) is an acid. We were physically attempting to help them blow off CO_2 in an effort to normalize their pH.

We were tracking this patient's ABGs—arterial blood gas—levels, through their arterial line, and they were hella acidotic. Normal pH ranges for an ABG are from 7.35-7.45. This patient was a 6.9 when I left right now. Long term and left unchecked, that's incompatible with life.

Other labs that were exceptionally bad—their potassium was 6.4 (normal's under 4.5), and their creatinine was nine-something (normal's under 1.3).

These are indicative of their kidneys being out of whack, which they were.

This patient was also almost thirty liters of fluid positive.

We pour fluids into people—we haven't even gotten into this patient's many, many, drips—and those fluids need to come out. Otherwise they're going to eventually wind up in the lungs, or the patient's going to swell up like Violet Beauregarde from Willy Wonka.

The reason we couldn't dialyze this patient (or more likely CRRT them) was because they were so unstable we couldn't even turn them over to put in the hemodialysis ports we'd have needed to take off some of that extra fluid.

They were proned, so that we could maximize their lung function from the jump, and they were so unstable subsequently that we were unable to ever flip them onto their back again. The fluid in their lungs would've sloshed around, filling up what functional tissue they did have, and they'd have died before they had the opportunity to gain anything from it.

And because we couldn't turn them without them dying, no one had changed the sheets out from underneath them. They had been on the same sheets for five days.

WHERE WAS that fluid coming from?

1) Levophed—a common blood pressure medication. Used to be called "leave 'em dead" because people used it for the sickest of the sick in sepsis and those patients still frequently died, but it has now come back into favor. We were maxed.

2) Vasopressin—another BP med. Not titratable. Left on normal dose.

3) Phenylephrine, aka Neo, from its brand name, Neosynephrine —another BP med—maxed. Pharmacy was mixing higher concentrations of this for us, so that we could give it in less fluid volume for the patient's sake.

4) Sodium Bicarb—also high-concentrated dose for fluid reasons —given to attempt to combat patient's acidosis.

5) Fentanyl—pain control—not maxed.

6) Versed—an amnesiac—hopefully makes you "less aware" of WTF is happening to you. Also not maxed, because they were also on....

7) Nimbex—a paralytic we give to patients to make them "ride the vent" so that they don't fight it and can save energy, as the vent does the work of breathing for them.

8) Heparin—blood thinner, to reduce the clotting that covid can cause.

9) Amiodarone—heart med, stops arrhythmias.

10) Insulin—which requires hourly insulin checks to titrate effectively. Unfortunately, many covid patients are also on steroids, which means their blood sugars fluctuate all over the place.

OUR GOAL with all of these was to keep the patient comfortable, riding the vent, completely unresponsive—intentionally—while we kept their systolic blood pressure above 90, and their MAP (mean arterial pressure) above 65.

Were we successful?

Fuck no.

This patient was a DNR, at least, which was good, because no one wanted to go into a code situation with someone this unstable. How can you give CPR to someone you can't even flip over?

We had no more tools left in our arsenal. There was, quite literally, nothing we could do for them.

The family didn't want to pull care, and I guess I get that, but like... it's just sad. Because there's no "there" there, anymore.

We did all the things we were supposed to, and it was a great learning experience for my proto-ICU-RN, but we were drawing labs knowing that there was nothing he could do about them. My trainee wanted to show our increasingly dire lab values to the Dr. and I had to pull her back and explain to her that it doesn't matter, and I very much promised he won't care. In fact, he might very well have laughed at her, as he was busy trying to keep people who had a chance at living alive, up the hall.

That patient's O_2 saturation was 66% when I left. Normal O_2 sats are from 95-100, and we usually aim for at least 92%. It had been trending down for hours. There was no setting we could go up to on the ventilator. I'm positive that patient had an anoxic brain injury. And their blood pressure was trending down the last few hours of my shift—same, same. Nothing we could do. Proceeding with care was futile.

I don't know if they'll be there when I go back to work tomorrow. I don't actually want them to be alive, for their sake. No one is coming back from a PEEP of 24. (Respiratory looked at their numbers in the morning and then looked at me and asked, "Do I really need to go in there?" and I was all, "Nope," and so they didn't.)

And we held all the bowel care medications we were supposed to give—which was A Lot of them, since the patient hadn't had a bowel movement yet during their stay. Narcotics constipate you, and paralytics can turn off normal peristalsis too. Do I want to make a patient who is very inevitably going to die, whom I have no way to turn over and clean thoroughly or effectively, shit themselves, costing them dignity in their final hours? No.

Which is to say I got as "comfort care-y" as I felt I could legally get.

This was definitely one of those situations where having visitors would've helped us—I think even in the abstract, over facetime, or hearing it from doctors, it's just too much for a family to process without seeing.

Anyhow—don't feel sorry for me, this is just another day at the office at this point. I just thought y'all would like to see how an average-to-busy day can roll and some of the behind-the-scenes thought processes I put in.

– Cassie

PS: They passed about three hours after we finished our shift.

———————————————————————————

1/29/21

We just had a body picked up by an inappropriately hot mortician. Apparently lifting dead bodies is a good workout.

It wasn't just me, all four of my coworkers in viewing range were all, "Whaaaaa????" And then after he left, one muttered, "who else can we kill?"

Don't judge, we've got to blow off steam somehow

Protestors block vaccination sites in Los Angeles. (1/30/21)

At some point in time during the prior month, Trump and his wife were vaccinated but did not tell anyone. (January 2021)

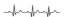

FEBRUARY 2021

2/1/21

This is my fifth 12-hr. shift in seven days, and the third of which I have trained new travel nurses.

2/1/21

Me, this morning, watching my traveler that I'm training pull out an old n95 to use from their backpack, because she thought we wouldn't have enough PPE: Darling, put that away and WELCOME TO CALIFORNIA.

2/2/21

Trying to figure out how much of this anxiety spiral I deserve because I'm clearly a bad person vs. just taking an Ativan and going the fuck to bed.

I know suffering isn't noble, I just actively have to deprogram myself from believing it two-four times a month.

I was really proud last night was a no meds night (although being dog tired from work helped.)

Apparently I didn't garden enough today, and I skipped rowing, thus leaving me with enough late-night energy to spin myself up.

2/3/21—password protected journal

Fuuuuuuck, y'all, I'm coming up on having lost a whole year of my life to this BS.

(And I know everyone has, it's just that this is my id-space to whine in right now, sorry.)

My birthday's next week. I'm going to be 45, which feels like a big number—we'd normally have a party for it; we usually celebrate the fives and zeroes big, you know?

But now, nothing.

This time last year I was in Cambria hanging out with my closest friends and now... I am not.

I haven't gotten to do ONE FUN THING THIS ENTIRE YEAR.

Since FOGcon last year, really. That convention was the weekend before I started working with covid patients and went into my own lockdown, and I have stayed there ever since.

I'm intensely responsible, but I definitely have that thrill-seeking, occasionally self-destructive gene in me that really needs to blow off steam.

And work's not helping. Work is fucking dull. Sad as hell, but dull as shit. We're not fighting fights we can win, so it's not scratching that itch, you know?

I have that feeling of fire ants inside my soul right now, where everything's just a jumble and all I want to do is let it out and... I can't. There's nowhere for it to go. There's nothing for it to do.

I can't lose myself at a show, or get a new tattoo. I can't even drive recklessly fast with the music blaring because there's nowhere for me to drive to! It's just all me and the ants and the ants are BORED, and I don't blame them because this past year has been the LONGEST YEAR I HAVE EVER LIVED.

I can't even go ride a fucking rollercoasterrrrrrr. (And covid took all my haunted houses away from me!)

Gah.

I volunteered to take care of covid patients the first day we had them—see: reckless, above—and now... the only thing different about them is the gradations of their sorrow.

I am so goddamned tired of being sad.

I want to be delighted. I want to be scared shitless. I want to be in lust. I want to be in pain—not emotional pain, or the pain of my relatives letting me down again—no, I want the crisp sharp pain of getting pierced, or of a needle driving ink beneath my skin. The kind where you hold yourself still before it happens and that's half of the delight, just seeing if you can. Like being in a fight before anyone throws a punch, but you know you're fucking in it and here it comes. Where you know it's going to hurt and you're going to be a little different on the other side.

That's what I want.

Feelings, again.

Clearly I kicked the wrong box inside my brain while writing earlier, and now it's like one of those "rattlesnake egg" gag gifts that won't stop whirring inside my mind.

And at least I know myself well enough that I know:

1. Yes, I'm like this, so these feelings aren't out or nowhere, nor are they a huge surprise; and
2. I'm not gonna go out and do anything stupid. (*Curse you, my responsible nature*)

But shiiiiit.

I would kill for a little genuine excitement.

Just something, anything, different, you know?

Bah.

Just got to tough it out.

But I totally understand the roaring '20s now, because if that was their reaction, post-war and post-1918 flu—yeah.

Once everyone gets vaxed and it's safe, I am going to be a hellion.

ALL OF THAT SAID...

Our covid numbers housewide are way down. From a high of 60 over the holidays to just hovering around 20 now, and only half of those are in the ICU. So we're making progress on that front, if only we can just keep people masked.

2/3/21—Two Nurses Talking newsletter

How I Get Back to "Normal," part one

Because someone asked....

CASSIE AGAIN!

Awhile back, we asked paid subscribers if there were any questions in particular they wanted answered, and someone asked how we got back to normal after shifts, and I thought I'd use this slot here to talk with y'all about how I do that that.

First off, "normal" is a very relative term, lol, so, uh, yeah. I've been nursing too long. I'm not even sure what my baseline is anymore.

But I do have a history of depression and anxiety, and whatever-the-fuck is happening to my brain due to covid isn't doing me any favors.

Luckily, I do know what to do when I get stressed—when I start feeling that gray and disconnected feeling, like the fog's starting to roll in.

Basically:

1) Get Social: Hang out with people in real life. It's hard with covid, but oddly work is good. Seeing my coworkers in real life 3-plus shifts a week super helps, especially because they understand.

2) Get Exercise: I have a rowing machine that I watch Netflix shows on, too. I just finished *The Untamed*, and now I'm halfway through *Hannibal*. I also do this class—L'agree fitness. If you ever want your ass kicked by an exercise class for an equivalent of crossfit, but which really does not injure your joints—and if you hate yourself very much, and want to torture yourself into the best shape of your life—L'agree is the modality for you. It's pricey as hell, but as someone who's had a ton of back injuries in my life and who has to keep using my back all the time at my job, I view these classes as an investment in keeping myself gainfully employed. I take my old studio's online classes at home now, using resistance bands and a pennyboard—a small skateboard—and sweet Jesus it is still terrorizing.

3) Get Outdoors: I garden.

A lot.

My frontyard/backyard gardening project began as my Trump Coping Memorial Garden back in 2016, when I couldn't handle how the world was going anymore. I started off with veggies, but found out that the way the sun goes over my house is too much for most of them.... and then I discovered the joy of succulents, especially this past year.

We did an earthquake retrofit awhile back and thought that we'd repanel on our own the room that the contractors destroyed, but then we didn't—so I reclaimed all that old redwood, plus assorted tables and chairs I've since picked up from the road in

Oakland, where I live, and freecycled all of the everything, basically. I have slowly bought, found, traded, and cultivated the plants.

What you are looking at is a... well, I wouldn't say World Class echeveria and succulent collection, because I'm pretty active on Instagram and I know there are people who're more intense than me, but I'm definitely above a hobbyist now. Maybe I'm semi-pro? Or semi-pro-pro-pro? Ha.

Here's my large echeveria variant section.

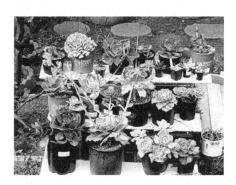

What's so cool is that these are all just different variations off of the same species of plant. Like all the different breeds of dogs, if you will.

I've also got an euphorbia section, a bromeliad section (with a ton of dyckia), a cactus zone, and all of the hanging succulents you might think of.

Gardening has been an especially useful hobby in covid times. It's relatively cheap because I find most of my structural elements roadside, dirt's cheap, and once you're tied into the succulent community it's pretty easy to find people to trade with online, or sellers to buy from. I'm also not afraid to get damaged plants at a discount, etc.

I'd like to claim I've got an amazing green thumb, but probably closer to the truth is that I live in zone 9b, which is just incredibly accommodating to succulents, although I do place shade cloth over my entire backyard each summer to stop my babies from getting sunburned.

So, yeah. When I start to lose myself, basically, I go outside. It turns out that taking meticulous care of living things that live is very spirit raising!

Y'all know I used to be a burn nurse, and a lot of being a burn nurse is enjoying picking at things—scabs, skin, taking out staples, that sort of ish—and I was telling another nurse at my new job that one of my favorite things to do is to pick off all the old leaves on my succulents—which is important! It stops them from getting bugs and helps prevent rot!—and she said, "That is the most ex-burn nurse thing I have ever heard," and laughed.

In closing, here's the world's most perfect echeveria orange sherbet (I'm pretty sure I've got that on lock):

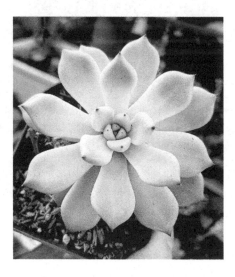

Coming up on Friday—thoughts about what normal really means for healthcare workers right now.

Until then!

– Cassie

2/3/21

I just want to have a taco Tuesday night again with my friends.

2/3/21

Wrote up my next Two Nurses Talking post today and make the mistake of opening up a brain box.

Hope is a bad thing, sometimes.

My birthday's next week and it's been a year of this shit, and 3/14, when all of this started for me, is coming up, and fair warning, I Will Be A Mess.

I just can't believe I've lost a year of my life to this. This is going to be my version of a midlife crisis, heh.

2/5/21—Two Nurses Talking newsletter

What is Normal, Anyways, for Nurses Right Now? Part two
   The "new" normal for HCW....

EVEN MORE CASSIE ;)

In going back and rereading the question that the subscriber asked (but after having already made my lovely plants post, because I love my plant-children)—and I kind of missed their point, so here goes on that—let me quote KB here:

My question is really basic, I guess. I want to know how you guys are doing. This is an invasive question, I know, but battlefield medics and doctors often have a hard time "reintegrating," for lack of a different word. And there's something about how the body reacts to long-term stress hormones. Do you think that the frontline workers as a whole are going to experience emotional and psychological issues when this is over? I don't see how you could avoid it. And if that occurs, how do you feel about the funding? Should there be a national program, federally funded, to help take care of the long-term effects to our frontline workers? I feel as though your heroic efforts to pull us through such a nightmare deserve at least that much. And so much more. Drinks for life, for sure.

On the whole....

You know how, when someone asks you how you're doing, and you say "Fine," because that's all you really want to share?

I say "Fine" a lot.

I find that, with the exception of what I consider to be somewhat therapeutic journaling here and elsewhere, and occasional pushes to get people to understand/behave, and flashes of anger because I want to yell—there's not much to be gained in discussing what's happening at the hospital with general civilians, even civilians that I consider to be friends. Even close friends. Even sometimes my husband. So don't take it personally.

Like the post I made earlier where I talked about my ten IV drips for that patient who was destined to die... some people were really horrified about that post and emailed me to make sure I was OK?

And I don't know how to deal with that, really.

I'm not telling you all stories here to have you sideline with me about my okayness, and honestly it weirds me out when you do, because that means you're clearly not okay with my level of okayness, and then I feel like there's an even wider gulf between me and normalcy.

Don't get me wrong, I love that people love me and worry about me, and I would do the same in your shoes, no doubt. It's just another weird level of strange, amplified by me not actually having a working framework within which to accept personal kindness. It's me, not you.

As I said at the bottom of that post....

These things now just have to be Another Day at The Office for me.

That's the only way I can continue to survive. Getting firehosed with loss and feelings would make doing my job impossible. If I sat around thinking about all the patients I've lost, in the abstract, or everything that I've lost—my ability to feel in discreet increments, for one—it just gets to be too much, so better never to think about it. At least for while, while we're still in the weeds.

I'm lucky because I only have to work three 12-hr. shifts a week to be full time at my job. That gives me four days to reset (see prior post, re: gardening) in a way that battlefield medics and military personnel don't. I'm even luckier that I can afford to live like that, and that I don't need to "cash out" right now. The temptation is certainly there, and I did more than my share earlier on, and I did far too many hours out of coworker solidarity in December....

But I am not the Saint of Being at the Hospital Because It Needs Me.

Do I still get three texts and emails a day, every day, begging me to go in?

Yes.

Do I feel bad about that?

Ehhhhhhhhhh.

I don't owe them or y'all shit, really.

I'm not a nurse because it's my magical calling, and in fact I don't think anyone is, or if you started like that, it gets totally burned out of you by the time you work your third year.

Sure, some moments still have magic in them, and I do hunt for those, for the strength to go on....

But it becomes increasingly obvious as This Continues that I Am Just Another Cog in The Machine and that my work satisfaction will be much better if I know my place.

This is about 40% because a ton of our covid patients die, so it's better for my brain somedays to not think about healing people, so much as pretending to be a strange, Ancient Egyptian-style goddess, whose job is to lead people to the underworld with as much peace and dignity as I can manage.

And it's about 60% because of the management at my hospital, who have, very aggressively, through assorted avenues (not the least of which is them dicking over our RT compatriots on their contracts at the end of last year) made it clear that we are all Replaceable and We Shouldn't Forget It.

It's hard to want to come in when there's no one in management who has your back.

And so my mental health is more important to me now. Plus, if I so much as look at a text from work about going in, my most excellent husband is all YOU ARE A WRITER, PUT THAT DOWN.

If you don't know, I write paranormal romance books. I actually became a nurse to be able to afford to live in the Bay Area and work part time so that I could write, because that's been my dream since I was like eight years old. See? Not a magical calling, but a means to an end.

It's that civilians thinking nursing is a "magical calling" bullshit that winds up with us being treated like "heroes" who should rise up to the moment to tolerate inhumane conditions for extraordinary periods of time.

Suffering is not noble. Neither my patients' suffering, nor mine.

So being less physically present at work helps, and even if it is crappy while I'm there, I'm able to fight to be normal more than most people who're there more frequently. And, frankly, I feel like I started off tougher than some, because having been a burn nurse prior was already its own kind of lonely.

You tell other nurses, even, that you're a burn nurse, and they're all, "Ooooh, I could never do that," and yeah, they're right, we're made of sterner stuff, but it's also a very ostracizing feeling.

Rather like being a garbage man, I imagine?

Because people aren't saying that shit because it's "hard" or "cool," like they might if I was claiming to be an astronaut. They're saying it because it's notoriously gross and they erroneously assume that it's sad.

So while sometimes I shared stories, generically, I hardly ever got to go into specifics, especially since the whys and hows of people getting burned are largely so personal, and I never wanted to out my patients. Also, there I got the chance to love my patients, because, by and large, they all survived. The job came with a satisfaction that few other nurses will ever really know, I think.

I would've crawled over glass for my manager on that unit. I could've devoted my life to that place, more than the ten years I gave it. I loved it so much, but my commute was so bad....

I TAKE WELLBUTRIN EVERY DAY, and Ativan and Ambien on an as-needed basis.

I suffer from depression, and Wellbutrin helps boost me out of the spiral. For me, it's been Good Stuff.

The Ativan is for my panic attacks, and, honestly, I probably don't take it often enough. I have that midwestern/Calvinist suffering streak where I think bootstraps are The Answer and that I should be endlessly tough. But fuck that, Ativan's great.

Same for Ambien. I try not to use it all the time, because I don't want to get too used to it, but sometimes I need it at night to turn my brain off.

I used to do therapy. [CA: I am very much back in therapy now.] I'm currently not sure what I'd say, other than the obvious, and I don't think there are any solutions for what's happening, seeing as it's situational, other than getting through it.

Also, as I've mentioned before, I compartmentalize the FUCK out of things (see my PTSD post earlier). Imagine a factory that makes boxes 24/7. That's my brain right now. It's like the warehouse side of an IKEA.

So oftentimes, I'm writing (and not all of my journals make it here) just to kind-of hold up a day or a memory or an experience and give it one nice shake before I fold it up and box it up forever.

I have a friend who is very good at remembering things, who has access to another place where I journal, even more messily, heh, and in the Before Times, she'd always ask me how I was doing, remembering a story I'd have written three weeks prior. She'd be all, "Whoa, that was pretty messed up—are you okay?"

And I'd be all, "Uh...which story was that again?"

And it wasn't that what happened, whatever I was journaling about, wasn't really bad at the time; generally the things were. It was just that I'd already boxed it up and put it away.

I would genuinely Not Remember.

And that's kind-of how I've always had to live my nursing life. I can't afford to remember all the sad shit I've seen, honestly. I gotta live my life, you know?

Is that healthy?

Well, kinda sorta.

It does build up, and if you box too fast, you lose track of your own feelings and your connection to reality becomes tenuous.

But I know that, so I fight to reconnect. I make sure to stay as active in other people's realities as I can handle.

I had a friend apologize to me yesterday for complaining about how messy her house was, because compared to my work.... and I was all, eff that, my house is a mess too; tell me more.

Because that's the world I long to get back to, the one where all we've got to complain about is having too much laundry to fold.

That's what I want. So badly.

I can't bring people into my life. It's too hard and sad—so what I want, I guess, is for them to bring me back to theirs. To remind me why going through all of this is worth it. So that I know that there's people who love me who're waiting somewhere on the other side, and if I just push long enough, I'll get to be there with them too.

One of the very last fun things I did last year pre-lockdown was a science fiction and fantasy author convention in early March, like the first weekend in March. And they're not going to have that again this year, obviously, so I'll have to wait for 2022.

But I have such a clear vision of what that'll involve when it gets to happen.

Me, sitting in the lobby like I always do, and people coming in and hugging me. I am not a Big Deal Author, but I like to think I'm Locally Well Known and Liked, and a lot of my writing community has held me particularly close this past year over assorted break downs elsewhere and in public on Twitter.

One of the things I enjoy about that community in particular, is that We All Seem to Share the Same Reality. All of my writer friends are taking this just as seriously as I am. They're masking, they're staying home, they're thinking ethically. I don't see photos of them online doing dumb shit to make this—the worst year of my life so far —last longer, tempting fate to infect their friends and family.

And because of that, I feel safe around them, which is why finally getting to take my armor off among them all will be okay.

So it'll be me, in the lobby, and everyone will come over and I'll probably start crying halfway through the first hug, and I may not stop all weekend long. I'll be so excited to see people again, to touch people again, all the people that I love and who've been rooting for me to make it through this—everyone who cheered when I got my vaccine—everyone who's seen all my dark nights of the soul on Twitter right before I wise up and take the Ativan.

I will get to be the messiest of mess people, just sobbing with Kleenex tucked up my sleeve like a grandma, and all of my friends who've seen me through this and whom I haven't had to worry about getting sick because they've all been so good, which I appreciate from the very bottom of my soul—we'll all be at the end of this very long, very dark, very awful tunnel, happily vaccinated, together.

I know it will happen.

I absolutely cannot wait.

I've been thinking about this particular scenario a lot, now that we're rounding the bend into spring. I drove into work early to volunteer to take care of covid patients on 3/14, not because I'm a good person, but because I'm a thrill seeker with a deathwish who is wired wrong. The good person part is beside the point. In an alternate reality I am a very happy rollercoaster engineer or something.

I will likely be having feelings next month, whether I like it or not. I'll see if I share some of them.

IN REGARD to HCW's mental wellbeing as a whole—yeah, we're fucked, we're all fucked, and we all know it.

Everyone I know is looking for a side-gig.

Even if the Biden administration turns things around, and I have great hopes for that, the psychological damage is done.

We were treated like garbage by the Trump administration. They stole our supplies and let our patients die and then made us watch it happen. They lied about what they were doing, they lied about masks, and they lied about drugs.

Everything we thought we knew as a profession, how we were treated, how we thought we were viewed by our communities, turned out to be bullshit.

The rug didn't just get pulled out from under us—they took the goddamned top three layers of soil with it, and left us to fall into the Earth's molten core.

I'm going to tough it out because I already have writing as a side-gig, which is occasionally lucrative, and I have managed to figure out some work-life balance.

But why would anyone else, who had any other options—going back to school, heading into tech/research, going into education, becoming a stay-at-home parent instead—keep working?

Will people be sad when they leave? Heck yeah.

But... after this past year... why on earth would you stay?

There'll be a fleet of young people coming in... possibly. I don't know. Would you want to sign on for what you just saw us do? When you could be a rollercoaster engineer instead? And that'll be great, and they'll replenish our ranks some, but they won't have the breadth nor depth of experience that older nurses do, and that brain drain's going to hurt hospitals badly.

As for ongoing psychological issues, oh, no doubt.

As for the government's ability to help us with those?

I laugh very hard at that and point to the dearth of programs for veterans of actual wars.

I think a lot of healthcare workers are just going to be deeply fucked up.

And they'll deal with that in different ways. Some will spend thousands of dollars and hours on a backyard-encompassing garden.... Others will start drinking, others will yell at their wives or do drugs....

I'm hoping that the rebound of freedom and normalcy at the end of this will help—kind of like the roaring '20s. I imagine there will be some epic parties and epic benders. Some of my most emotionally healing moments have been while I was intensely altered, hanging out with my closest friends, and I would dearly like to get to have those opportunities again. To fall and be caught by those who love you is a really good feeling, you know?

I suspect it'll reprioritize a lot of people's lives, having been so close to death for so long—people are going to want to do things that are important to them, and not put anything off ever again, and more power to them. I'm a big proponent of living your life as authentically as you can. And harm none, do what ye will and all that.

But I don't actually want drinks for life, and after a while I don't think I'll ever want to talk about all this that much again.

Wallowing's not healthy. As a former burn nurse—I know that to be healthy you've got to make sure you only pick the right scabs.

I get now why people say their grandfathers never talked about the war, because the experiential gulf of having been in the trenches versus having a conversation with someone who wasn't there and can't contextualize the moment is almost insurmountable.

It's fucking hard for me to explain to you here—and I'm a writer!

And then my writing evokes your feelings, which is great, that's its job, but I don't really want those feelings pointed at me.

I don't want people going through life thinking I'm wounded because of all of this, even though that might partially be the case. I am tired of being strange, and there will come a time when I don't want to talk about anymore having been strange, because it is exhausting.

I don't want people thinking they need to treat me differently, and I definitely do not want your pity, and at this stage in my atheism game I'm frankly insulted by your prayers—because if God exists this certainly is SOME BULLSHIT, NO?

So when all of this is said and done, I just really want to go back to being normal.

I want to live my life again—just like all of you do, I'm sure.

I want to wander around garden centers aimlessly and buy plants I almost certainly do not need.

I want to go out to dinner with my girlfriends and laugh until I snort.

I want to take drives that actually go somewhere, like on trips, away from my house.

I want to go on so many writing retreats!

I want to go on hikes, and get pedicures, and hang out at coffee shops both with and without friends.

I want to see other people's smiles again.

I want to go dancing—and I want to see shows. So many shows! I tell you, after this, I will never, ever, skip a show I want to see, ever again in my life.

So, yeah—I don't want this episode to be the sum total of who I am, even if it may be the reason you currently know me. I want there to be more to me than just this, and I don't want to be anchored by this event in the future either, if that makes sense.

When this is the past—and we will get there, even though it'll take time—I want it to be in my past, too.

This version of me that I'm being forced to be now is not truly who I am. But I have great hopes for the version of me that I get to be in the future.

Just got to get there, is all.

– Cassie

Texas Congressman Ron Wright dies of covid after having made it a political football. (2/8/21)

2/8/21

I hope this dude and Herman Cain are high fiving in hell right now.

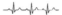

THIS TWEET in particular seems to have set certain people off, and I'd just like to address that type of thing right now again, here.

To those people who think we need to "respect the dead" above all else—if you were advocating for pro-covid policies when you were alive, thus enabling it to kill other people, before, SURPRISE, it got you, too... yeah, fuck you.

I don't feel bad in the least for making fun of this dude, or Herman Cain (whose Twitter account, some of you will remember, continued to post pro-Trump content, even after he died—from having gotten covid at a Trump rally!)

At this point in time, I had spent almost a whole year of my life easing people into the ground—so no.

I'll respect my dead patients, yes.

I'll take out all their lines, wash their bodies down with warm wipes, and cross their arms across their chest after I put them into a body bag.

But if you've never put someone into a body bag, don't you come for me, thinking you can BEGIN to talk to me ABOUT DEAD PEOPLE.

Not in this lifetime, nor in the next.

.   .   .

OH, and, I forgot, some guy was hounding me after this tweet, saying stuff like he hoped I went to hell.

First off, I don't believe in hell, because why would God punish people for things that are essentially out of their control?

Secondly, as I told him back, my dude—if there is a hell, I've already been there.

What could be worse, more emotionally painful, more morally depressing, than what I and four million other nurses went through last year?

How puerile to think that hell exists because God needs an entirely separate way to torture us later, when He has so many here on Earth?

2/9/21

The other day when I was warning about feeing emotionally barfy, and y'all all were like, "We've got you," well—you were right. I had such a good birthday, y'all, and half of the reason for that was because I asked for love and I got it.

Lessons were learned.

It's real hard to flip the switch and take off the armor.

I remember when I used to go into work, driving in the dark, into my 11p nightshift, and all I could think about was putting the armor on that I needed in order to be a baby nurse....

Little did I know it would become a part of me and that a day would come when I wouldn't be able to take it off without peeling away skin. And covid this past year has effing steam-ironed that shit on tight.

So I'm really glad I asked for love and got it, on all sorts of fronts.

And on Friday, my husband got let go from his job (because they're stupid, basically) and that was just adding to all the Life Stress. But he reached out to people as well, and his friends were all, "Lolwut? send me your resume posthaste," and he's already gotten five job offers.

And we were just kind-of marveling a bit ago at how lucky both of us are. I think we vastly underestimated how much other people want to help and love on other people who they love, especially in this strange, weird time.

And that while it's good to be tough, try not to be so tough that you can't let other people help you.

People want to help you, if you can slow down long enough to let them in.

It's nice to know that there's goodness waiting in the wings.

I don't want to sound Pollyanna, and I so, so know life is essentially unfair.

But a small part of my soul was restored by assorted kindnesses thrust upon me and mine this past weekend, and I needed that.

2/10/21

Past me signed me up to work six outta eight days here, like a real jerk.

2/10/21

Today at work is kicking my ass, in a good way. One patient had covid back in June, left, and is now back to die. But my other might actually live? As long as I can keep their brain where it's supposed to be, heh. And our covid numbers are way, way down!

2/11/21

Just doing my best today to provide that Quality Death Experience (tm).

2/11/21

So the palliative care MD came up to me, and I thought it was re: my currently dying patient, but no.

A family from a death I'd overseen three months ago was on the phone and asking her questions. Picking apart what they'd seen me say and do in the room on facetime at the end.

And I, as always, but especially when death is on the line —*Princess Bride* reference intentional—had been giving my A game.

But what do they know?

How many people have they seen die?

More importantly... how many deaths do they know they've caused?

Because that's what it was really about. Someone in their family killed someone else with covid. And now the survivors are all sitting at home, stewing, hurting, looking anywhere else they can to place blame.

When I heard they'd been second guessing me it was like a gut punch. I wanted to cry. Didn't they know I'd tried my hardest? Didn't they see me crying, too?

But I know it's not about me. It's about them, just desperately trying to figure a way out of the cage they locked themselves in. The one where they know they gave someone they loved covid. And that person died.

There's going to be so many people so fucked up at the end of this, y'all.

At least when I kill people, via comfort care, or by

watching them not manage to survive no matter what interventions we do, I get to live clean at night.

It hurts, it's awful, it's too much—but I'm only there for the end. I know I never *started* shit.

If you're tired of masking, tired of not partying, tired of not seeing grandma—just think about what it'd be like to live the rest of your life knowing you killed someone you loved.

⎍⎍⎍⎍⎍

I UNDERSTOOD why they were asking, because sitting at home with the knowledge that you killed someone you loved—because everyone who got covid got it from someone else—is surely *too much*... but at the same time, I am a human, too. Not some care-giving robot.

I didn't give up on your loved one. You just asked me to do the impossible.

I couldn't.

But I freaking tried.

⎍⎍⎍⎍⎍

President Biden announces that enough vaccines have been procured for the entire United States to be vaccinated by the end of July. (2/11/21)

⎍⎍⎍⎍⎍

2/11/2021—password protected journal

Y'ALL BIDEN SAID THEY'VE PROCURED ENOUGH VAX FOR THE ENTIRE USA TO BE VAXED BY THE END OF JULY.

I need this to work out logistically SO HARD.

That's just five months away!!!!

And like, as things start rolling out, numbers will be getting better and better, and YYYEEESSSSS.

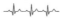

2/12/21—Two Nurses Talking newsletter

Admiral Ackbar's Geranium

Yes, that Admiral Ackbar.

THIS IS A 100% true story—but let me preface this by saying I don't actually like geraniums.

I love a ton of plants, but geraniums don't do it for me—I don't have the patience to deadhead them when I'm supposed to so they always wind up looking scraggly.

But I still have a bunch in my front yard, from this home's prior owner. I had my gardeners cut them back when I was going All Succulent All the Time...but the effers grew back anyways. Around my succulents. So now there's a whole hostage situation going on, where I can't water one without watering the others, and on some level, I have to respect that.

You've heard me talk here before about the imminent brain drain that'll happen when as many of us as can escape bedside nursing do so post-covid, but I realized I never really gave you an example of what that means, so here goes.

This one just happens to involve a famous person.

A few years ago, I was hanging out with one of my writing besties in Berkeley.

She and her husband were the on-site managers of an apartment complex. It was brutalist-style, all cement, and apparently it was the reason they redid zoning laws in Berkeley to not allow buildings over a certain height, as the structure was quite ugly.

The whole complex was locked, though, and we were hanging out, as we so often did, in her living room, with the sliding glass door opened on one side to her small balcony full of plants, and the door to the rest of the complex open to the shared hallway—just desperately trying to catch a breeze.

We were writing together and then had plans to go into San Francisco that evening—when one of her neighbors came by.

He was an older man, talking about how his internet wasn't working, and asking her what she could do to fix it. He walked right on into her apartment, through the open door, and something was off.

First off, he was complaining about how he wouldn't be able to get jobs if his internet didn't work, which made sense, but... he was so old. I was wondering if he really had to work.... (Nurses are nosy as fuck.) And while he was kempt, it was an -ish situation. I could tell he wasn't 100% okay. There was something about the way he was walking, stalking back and forth inside her apartment, and the way he said his phrases, angrily demanding satisfaction from her—I wasn't scared, but I could feel my Something's Not Right Here nursing alarms going off inside my head.

After my friend had explained to him that he'd have to call his internet service provider to figure things out, and he'd left, she turned to me and said, "Yeah, he just came back from the hospital for dehydration."

My next thought was, "Goddammit, *fuck me.*"

I curse in real life as often as I do on here. And I think that particular phrase often, anytime things seem like they're going in an unfair direction—or when I'm being placed in an unwanted position to be the one to Do Something, whether I'm interested in that or not.

Because as a nurse I happen to know that elderly people get dehydrated easily, and that if your electrolytes get off—particularly with sodium—you'll start to act funny, because it messes with your brain.

I can't ignore it, it's not in my nature, so we walk down to his apartment, which is open in a similar fashion to hers, to at least do a wellness check. We walk right on into his place, and I notice it's nicely kept up, and he does have a lot of awards related to voice acting on his bookshelves and plaques on his walls. But he's still being... him.

Not right. Talking wrong—not 100% wrong, but 20% wrong, the kind of wrong you've got to listen to for a while to realize that it's off. I pull out my phone and call 911, and we hang out with him, him still complaining all the while about his internet, as the firetruck pulls in.

Berkeley Fire is really uninterested in trusting my nursing abilities.

And I don't blame them. I used to do hospital transfers, and I know EMS is always busy and they see a lot of shit.

And it doesn't help that he's complaining, vociferously, that he doesn't want them there.

In 911-land, if someone doesn't want you to give them care, they have to honor that.

They won't.

They'll wait for your dumbass to pass out and then they'll start doing CPR or intubate you or whatever else is appropriate for your care.

So this guy's all, "Get out of my apartment!" And they're all, "Sure, gramps," ready to turn tail, and I'm all, "No. I am a nurse. This man needs to be hospitalized. He was just hospitalized for dehydration and it's happening again, I'm sure."

I make them wait there and talk him into at least a vitals check—and by the end of that five-minute period, their spidey-senses are tingling too. Even though his vitals are normal.

Once the paramedic agrees with me, and they strap him on a gurney to take him in against his wishes. My friend calls the man's emergency contact to let him know he's going back into the hospital, and we grab our stuff to head into the city.

Halfway out to my car she looks over at me. "You know that guy —he's Admiral Ackbar."

And I'm all, "Huh?"

"The guy that says, 'It's a trap!' in the Star Wars films—that's him."

And I'm all, "Whhhhhhhaaaaatttttt...." But suddenly all the voice acting awards he'd had on his walls made sense.

We go on and have our evening in SF together, and I drop her off afterwards, and she asks me how I think he'll do, and I say, "Probably not good," because if you live alone and you're not getting your intrinsic kick to drink at appropriate times, well, you're going to become dysregulated if there's no one else around to do it for you.

And sure enough, a few weeks later, he winds up passing.

He also, like my friend, had a balcony with plants—and his care-taker friend (who didn't live with him, but who helped him manage his affairs) gave my friend several of them.

And she gave his geranium to me.

So this is Admiral Ackbar's geranium:

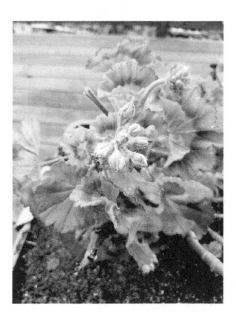

Which is now the one geranium I'm absolutely not allowed to kill, although I haven't always treated it gently. (In this photo, I have just repotted it into a much, much bigger pot, so that it can take up a prime spot on my deck.)

Whatever it is that I did for that man?

New nurses don't have that.

Some of it is the breadth of experience—some nursing events you just need to live through, for that experience to sink in—and some of that is gumption. The strength to do the right thing and be bossy when needed. My friend knew no better, and 911 wouldn't have cared if I hadn't bullied them into caring.

He'd have just slipped through the cracks.

You might think, if you're a HCW yourself, that that's kind of an easy catch, and maybe it is, but it's the easiest way for me to explain what it's like to be a nurse moving through the world.

Because I can't explain what it's like to just walk into the room, look at someone's positioning in their bed and their color and just know that things are wrong. That ominous sense you get when someone's about to go septic on you. That pressurized lull before the storm when you say, "get the crash cart."

Maybe it's like being a mom? I don't know; I don't have kids, so I can't speak to that.

All I do know is that I can walk into a room at work, and if God wants you to live today, I can get you there. But sometimes those extra seconds that my spidey-sense buys you—and my willingness to stare down other providers and get you the attention you need, fearlessly escalating if I have too, when other people are looking at numbers on screens but not seeing you, touching you, smelling you, like I am—that shit counts.

And that's what's walking out the door, after all of this—to other jobs, or early retirement. You can't blame us; we're tired and sad and we've all got PTSD. There's just going to be a gap of a few years in there, post-covid-times, where you shouldn't trust any nurse that's too excited to be working.

They'll mean well, but they won't know anything.
– Cassie

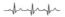

2/12/21

I thought I would feel more feels watching *The Stand*, due to pandemic reasons, but honestly the good vs evil conflict feels depressingly dated now that we've all been exposed to a firehose of banal evil and selfishness this past year.

2/14/21

There's not much that makes me cringe at work, except for replacing a condom cath for the fourth time.

I'm just tired of touching this guy's dick. (I got a guy to go in there and do it last time.)

Like once you can chat through. Twice, yeah. By the fourth time you're all THERE IS NO SMALL TALK THAT CAN OVERCOME THIS.

I must now be a machine of dick-touching efficiency. Pay no attention to the hands on your junk.

It is my least favorite thing to do, off of a very long roster of unfavorite things, that includes such stellar options as: getting shit out of vaginas and suctioning nasal mucus.

Just helped to clean a GI-bleed shit with so much blood in it you could taste the tang of iron while cleaning.

2/15/21—Two Nurses Talking newsletter

The Art of Saying Nothing
Because sometimes there's nothing you can say.

I STARTED off with a very short career in sales before I went to nursing school. This was before AirBnB was a thing—the place I worked for had a business model based around renting out people's unused vacation homes in Cabo San Lucas. There were twenty of us in the office, and we all worked for one rich guy who had several homes himself.

It was an interesting experience—I doubt they're still around now —and it taught me a lot about how to be circumspect.

You see I'd never been to Cabo, personally.

We had a DOS program, where you'd put in how many rooms people needed, and the dates, and we could go off of available inventory, figuring things out—and there were photos I could look at, which I could send to the clients, online.

But I didn't really know anything.

I just sounded really good on the phone.

I learned very early on that people who're about to go on vacation —and oftentimes spend A Ton of Money on Vacation—are very anxious, especially when they've never been to their destinations, etc. And I was their tour guide, in a way. I could make recommendations for nearby restaurants, from which I'm sure our owner got a kickback; I knew which beaches were safe to swim at, and which were not, etc. We rented homes to some very famous people, and in one memorable escapade had Someone Famous break a glass coffee table that we had to replace because they were drunk off their ass in one of these houses.

My job was to sell these rentals, yes, but also to not oversell them. It didn't do my boss nor me any favors since I got paid on commission, to hype things that couldn't happen or make promises that I couldn't execute on.

Because there's nothing worse than disappointment, right?

And I think about that training experience a lot now, as a covid nurse.

FAMILY CALLS.

They want to know if their loved one is better.

I always, always, always ask when they were last updated. Usually it's been within 24 hours, and oftentimes I can say "nothing's changed," if that's true.

Then they want me to read them the vitals off the monitor or the ventilator, and major lab values, if their loved one's been in the hospital awhile, and we've been explaining things along the way.

You just always have to be so careful about not hyping anything up, ever, and you have to contextualize everything, all the time.

Sure, they may be on a little less oxygen today, percentagewise, but, you know, going from 80% to 75% isn't all that great a change, seeing as you're not extubatable till you're down to 40% or less.

Or their PEEP might be better, but that could be because we've got them on their stomach, and seeing as how you can't live on your stomach, that's not real helpful.

SOMETIMES I FEEL like a cruel nanny—like the family member is a toddler, and all they want to do is to run out an open door. They can see hope through the doorframe, and all they've got to do is get past me to get out into it.

But I can't let them do that. It's not fair to them, expectation-wise, and it's not therapeutic for the patient—if you're basing Big Decisions off of how they're doing, if our palliative care team is having Goals of Care talks with you—I can't even let you see a glimmer of a pipe dream.

Any hope I offer has to come utterly tethered to reality.

So family members will fish, as I box and try to lower expectations, and somedays—most days—the best thing I can offer is, "They're not getting better—but they're also not getting worse." Or, "We're giving them a chance to heal. We just have to see if they can take it."

I know that hurts on the other end of the line. Especially with covid, man, because it can be such a yo-yo—people really can be doing better, and then their lungs punk out, and it's such a "two steps forward, three steps back" disease.

I don't like having these sorts of conversations—basically, any time you need to tell a family member "these injuries are incompatible with life," it's a huge bummer. And I know that it makes me seem like a dick, and some people get really frustrated—but it's really the only ethical way for me to present the scenario.

I would so much rather a patient prove me wrong by going on to do unexpectedly better than surmised, than have a family member sobbing because a death came out of left field.

I can take the occasional and occasionally snide, "They sure proved you wrong, didn't they?" so much better than, "But everything was going fine, you said so!"

IT IS a rough time to be in a profession where you can't give people exactly what they want.

If covid has made anything clear to us, it is that in the wider world, the general American population expects The Customer to Be Always Right, even when the topics are as important as the utility of masks and the timing of restaurant reopenings. And now that everyone's become an armchair epidemiologist....

But I can't give that message to people at work, you know? I can't fix lungs. I can't make things "right." I can only report honestly on what I'm seeing, and what experience has led me to predict the path will be.

So I've gotten very good at saying nothing at all—nothing positive, at least—when giving information, not to protect myself, but to protect the family's expectations.

I CAN'T OVERSELL the condo. The view's bleak, there's sharks in the water, and there's not enough air.

– Cassie

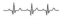

2/17/21—Two Nurses Talking newsletter

I Hope You're Not My Nurse!
(i.e., Will you still do CPR on me if I'm Republican?)

PEOPLE ON TWITTER say this to me ALL THE TIME when I brawl about masks and hypocrisy.

Like they think they're going to hurt my feelings.

Newsflash asshat: I DON'T WANT TO BE YOUR NURSE.

How daft must these people be, to think that's some kind of insult?

Like I'm going to weep gently at night... not taking care of them?

Guess what? It turns out I genuinely DO NOT WANT YOU TO GET COVID.

That is why I'm on this Twitter thread TRYING TO POINT OUT PUBLIC HEALTH GUIDELINES.

I mean, go ahead man, don't wear a mask, breathe other people's air, prove me wrong if you gotta, but... sheesh?

These people are always closely followed by the, "I bet your quality of care is less based on politics!"

That's actually a valid question, so let me get into that.

First off, no, and I'm horrified you'd ask that, although if I'm being angry on Twitter, I can understand your reasons for concern, but....

I'm a liberal softy. I generally just want to give you free health care and college, based on taxing the 0.0001% richest people in America.

In fact, the only reason I'm yelling at you and yours on Twitter is BECAUSE YOU ARE TRYING TO KILL PEOPLE WITH YOUR ASSHATTERY.

If you weren't, you wouldn't even know my name! Nor I, yours!

If you're reading this now, and you've made it this far, because I sent you this link on Twitter so that you can read my summary of my attitudes about the subject, I'd encourage you to read some more articles on this site.

At work I have been punched, kicked, spit on, and had food and bodily wastes thrown at me. I have had to watch people die who didn't have to, and probably watched some people die who deserved it, although I didn't know it at the time.

Invariably, despite of all that violence directed against me, emotionally, mentally, and physically, I have always given ALL OF THOSE PATIENTS my A-game.

Why?

Because I take pride in what I do.

And?

At the end, when you're holding someone's life in your hands, even if they're a shitbird, they're still so vastly, terribly, terrifically human.

I don't want to get misty-eyed about getting spat at, but usually, when people are doing that shit?

They're broken.

Something in their head, or their lives, or in the system, has horribly let them down.

At the end of my shift, I get to leave my job and come home to my husband and my cat.

Normal people aren't throwing shit or throwing punches, you know?

So even though I don't enjoy those altercations with those people, I'm not going to give them worse care. Something happened to them —something bad.

I'll take safety precautions, heck yes, and get other RNs to watch my back if shit gets rough, but I'm not going to hold out meds or care on someone like that—fuck no. If you're acting up like that, chances are you REALLY NEED THEM.

There was a part in one of my books I wrote recently, with my coauthor, wherein the nurse protag did something to help a bad guy, and my coauthor was all, "Whoa, would she really do that?"

And I was all, "Uh, yeah, of course she would."

At the time, the example I used was of Donald Trump needing CPR.

Would I be happy about giving it to him?

No.

But would I do it if I had too?

Yes.

Cussing and yelling all the time, but I'd still be giving good compressions and allowing for chest recoil.

The only, only, only, only time I have ever been even the teeniest bit bad was when I worked at the burn unit and this guy came in with a huge Nazi tattoo that'd gotten burned. I may have scrubbed it a little harder, just in case...but the burns were superficial, and it didn't come off.

So here we go: I've written it in stone now, for all my past, present, and future Twitter haters, so I can send them this link—NO, I NEVER WANT TO BE YOUR NURSE.

But if I had to be?

You'd be OK. I'd make sure of it.

Maybe stop yelling at me and wear a mask?

Love,

– Cassie

2/18/21

Overheard in the ED (where I still am), "like what dollar amount of cocaine do you use a week?"

"Hundred."

"Yeah, that's bad for your kidneys. Stop."

2/19/21

Lol, my biodad getting saucy in an email—he saves these bon mots up for me and then rants about once a week—regarding Rush Limbaugh dying: "America no longer has its colostomy bag."

2/21/21

Our number is just a handful here today, y'all. I can't tell you how different the mood is with so few covid cases.

We're well aware this is like a microclimate thing, in that the Bay is doing well. I know shit's still hard elsewhere.

Still, feels like exhaling.

2/21/2021—password protected journal

Down to just five covid patients at my hospital!!!!!

From a high of half our beds this winter!

And now friends of mine who are teachers are getting vaccinated, and it's just feeling more real/possible/plausible now.

Apparently another nearby hospital is still busy—and we're still seeing patients who got over covid earlier in the year come back through—but but but...

Just five.

2/22/21

One thing I am very much looking forward to leaving behind in this quarantine is the high-pressure world of men's haircuts.

2/23/21

If you qualify for a vaccine in any way, shape, or form, and you're the least bit hesitant about getting it, please don't be.

I can officially absolve you of guilt if you'd like.

Please, please, please take your turn when its offered, and if people judge you, send 'em my way for yell-time.

2/25/2021—password protected journal

I hung out, outside, masked, with E on Tues, and then same-same with V on Weds!

I feel like I've got to build my capacity for these sorts of things back up in small ways—it's so funny, like a day where I do two errands feels IMPOSSIBLE, which is dumb, because back in the day I was a three-four errand/hang a day girl, heh. (In general, I have been a no-errands-any-day person for lo these many moons now.)

But it's been really good to see people in person this past week :D :D :D

Feels like the ice is thawing and normal's just around the corner.

2/26/21

YOU ALL, I HAVE GOOD NEWS! LISTEN UP. There are no covid cases in my ICU today!!!!!!!!!!! Just a handful house-wide but NONE HERE!!!!!

2/27/21

...waiting on the covid test for my upcoming admit with shortness of breath and a shitty x-ray.

2/27/21

People who've had covid and don't want bad news, look away —people who're tempted to unmask or need more encouragement to make it through these final few months, listen up.

So my "maybe covid" patient this morning—I'm n95ing up, and we're treating them like covid till I hear otherwise. The reason I'm gowning up is that, even though the fast test was negative, their x-rays show lung damage akin to covid, so we're playing it safe while we do a send-out test.

Well, a relative just dropped off some goodies for them and I went down to pick them up in person.

Turns out everyone in their house had covid in November. Why this didn't come up earlier, via paramedics or ED staff, or in the chart, I don't know.

When I mentioned their not-great x-rays, the family member was all, "But it didn't feel respiratory at the time."

That's how it gets you, man. And how many people who blew it off, or didn't and still caught it, have damage they don't know about yet?

That they won't know about until another medical issue arises and compounds things?

Keep your masks on tight.

2/28/21

I don't want to be your hero, I want retroactive hazard pay and future mental health care.

OH, AND STUDENT LOAN FORGIVENESS, which is literally the LEAST you could do.

(That would be too late to help me, but loans are a yoke around so many younger RNs.)

[CA: in response to Amy Klobuchar, Minnesota Senator, tweeting that 'Nurses are heroes.']

2/28/21

There's an art to keeping an eye on your fidgety patient who took out their central line while you were on break—got to come back to a bed full of blood, hooray!—and staying out of sight enough to not be being called into the room for anxious nonsense.

2/28/21

Had kind of a profound realization here at work just now.

I hate working three-day stretches because I can keep you alive day three, but I can't be nice.

And honestly, it's been hard to be nice to patients for months now. Nursing real talk zone here, so take your hero bullshit elsewhere.

It's because for so long I've had to just think about patients as meat sacks... or complicated instruments that I knew how to play.

Because being too kind wound up just hurting harder.

Over and over again. I lost faith in kindness because it did nothing but burn me.

Anyhow, today I was trying to figure out how to get that back, you know? Especially when I'm still taking care of dying people, alas, albeit for non-covid reasons. I was wondering if there'd be a switch or something, you know? Or a health bar like in a videogame.

I was just kind of assuming one day I'd wake up and my kindness well would be refilled.

But then today, I was with my very, very sick patient, who is 100% going to die in a lingering horrible way thru no fault of their own, in one of those "life support does not equal the ability to live without ICU-shit" kind of ways, which is soul grinding on own.

I was all, "Fuck it. End of day three. Let's get back on this niceness wagon. We have a few days off after this to recoup, so it's okay if it hurts, again, like we know it will, again." So I slam a Coke Zero and dredge up some empathy to share.

And afterwards I'm all, "Yeah! I did that!"

And? It didn't even hurt.

I mean... it changes nothing in the grand scheme, care-wise.

Death is death and it certainly comes for us all.

But I got a little piece of my soul back.

And my work kindness health bar us like 5% refilled. Kindness begets kindness, and the secret to finding it again was just being brave enough to try doing it again.

And so here I am crying on break in the old family waiting room. (I'm going to really miss this lovely window-filled space when visitors come back, heh.) Phew.

I'm sure this sounds super simple/obvious to y'all, like, duh, but it's been... so long since it's been safe. There's still a lot of my health bar to refill. And I might backslide some, now that I have to think about it, because it's not instinct.

But maybe, just maybe, I'm going to be okay. Eventually. At least I know how to fake it till you make it, as always.

MARCH 2021

One of my prized plants is dying.

I am more messed up about this than I ought to be.

I can't tell if it's PMS or just the end of my rope when I can't save one beautiful, quality thing that I love and have loved for years, so fuck it all.

I think it's just going to be like this for a while. Like I'll think I'm good and over stuff and I've got this mental health thing figured out, and PTSD-schmee-TSD, and then, *surprise!* I accidentally open a box and get to feel feelings, and suddenly inexorably losing a plant that I love is clearly indicative of all the people I've had to watch die over the past 12 months and shit sucks, and I'm doing the kind of guttyworks crying usually reserved for the death of a pet and asking my husband to lay on top of me like a human weighted blanket and/or squeeze machine until I can figure out which way all the pieces fit into the goddamned box again and put the lid back on.

I just have to accept that the buffer between me and mental wellness is waxing and waning all the time, like a set of lungs I have no control over breathing.

At no point in time will I ever have it on lock.

Governor Abbott of Texas lifts mask mandate, 100%, statewide. (3/2/21)

3/2/21

I think part of the reason my brain's been yo-yoing so hard lately, in addition to the anniversary of all this shit, is that covid's made it patently clear that decisions made nationwide affect all of us.

So while news in CA is great right now, numbers down, pumping vax into people, A+++, watching other states make grim decisions and sacrificing their populace for nothing.... It just still is heart rendering.

I can't be all, "Oh, whatevs, it's in some other state."

Those nurses there have been living in a meatgrinder I know all too well, and to just see them chopped up and fed through for another pass, on top of the inevitable loss of human life now and later....

Haven't we learned ANYTHING yet? ANYTHING AT ALL?

It's just so dispiriting. I suspect the answer is to look away, but I can't. It's my relatives, and buddies from high school, since I grew up in TX, and it's my freaking profession to look at the bad... to prepare myself to deal with it and try to get out ahead of it.

It's just the sabotage of it all, when we all know better by now, by all the science, by every metric. It's like an entire state is subject to Lucy yanking the ball away from Charlie Brown, only people will die or find out their lungs suck later, entirely due to @GovAbbott .

His ass is vaccinated. My friends and relatives are not.

Eff you, Abbott.

You announcing killing people like you're proud of it.

I'd ask what kind of government that is, but I already know.

3/4/21

I'm going have to take a post-OP covid patient in two hours, thus breaking our ICU's lovely No Covid Patients stretch.

kicks a rock

Whelp, my post-op covid got bumped (still coming up, but for someone else, later) by someone on 100% high flow, for us to manually prone. I bought my "feeling sorry for myself" Snickers and KitKat, as is my wont.

I won't lie; I'm fucking bummed. I don't mind taking care of covid pts, but I foolishly hoped we were done. House-wide numbers were slowly scooting up though, so someone getting sicker was inevitable.

My coworker just now, exceedingly dryly (as all ICU humor is), "I hear covid doesn't exist in Texas, so maybe we can transfer them."

Newsflash: My admit doesn't have active covid... and they've been here so long they're not in isolation anymore. They're in that elliptical "trapped in the hospital with trashed lungs" orbit, and can't achieve escape velocity. So yay for me. Not so much for them.

3/4/21 - later

Finally coming down from how wired I got at work, with the help of a Netflix-party *Voyager* watching and a pint of B&J's.

I think this is the new long-haul, for health care workers: People who aren't dying of active covid, but who can't escape the yawning maw of its grasp.

My patient on the high-flow landed and crashed. Intubated, arterial line, central line, foley, oral-gastric tube, propofol, fentanyl, and I'm sure they'll be nimbexed (paralyzed) and proned overnight, if they live that long.

Their scared eyes, knowing what's coming, because they've been in that exact same position—in our exact same hospital—before. Just weeks ago.

It is something else, watching someone's oxygenation numbers dropping when they try to talk to you.

It is also something else taking away someone's phone because their only job is breathing, no distractions, we mean it. Just breathe, please, breathe.

Flipping them over in case it does anything. Watching them pant like a dog.

Their ABG was 7.6. That's hella alkalotic, for people who don't know that shit. CO_2's an acid, and they were breathing all of theirs off. That's when we flipped 'em back and said, "You want this?" and started in.

Maybe that phone call I didn't let them take would've been the last time they could've talked to someone.

But I couldn't take the chance, since they weren't breathing enough as it was.

Shit's fucked.

[CA: this patient died a month later and was never able to speak again in the interim. I am haunted by this, now.]

—⅃⅄⅃⅄—

3/4/21

Luckily this ridiculous tortie beast loves me very much. (For people sending virtual hugs/cats, this is me in real life right now, heh.)

[CA: not shown, photo of Milly on my chest.]

3/5/21

Every time I can't log into Epic, I assume I've been fired.

[CA: Epic is our charting program at work.}

Coworker's patient got tPA and forgot they'd had very recent dental work, so now they're drooling blood like a zombie.

[CA: tPA is a clot-busting blood thinner.]

3/6/21

Some people go to therapy, other people pre-schedule 3700-word newsletter posts. Same diff, really.

3/10/21—Two Nurses Talking newsletter

Back to Just Normal Dying.

CW: death, obviously

CASSIE here again (and I've prescheduled some posts and L is on vacation soon, so the next few will likely be from me, too.)

Had my first real interaction with a family under non-covid circumstances yesterday.

They were only allowed to visit because their loved one was dying, and our visitation procedures are still really hardcore... but eventually there were four strangers in the room with me, along with their loved one.

It's been so very, very long since I've seen a "normal" death that I'd almost forgotten what to do.

When covid patients died... you didn't get a choice. They were on that freaking train, and it was coming into station. Things always felt fast, even when they weren't, with very few exceptions.

But this was a death of a more leisurely sort. The kind where you get the chance to hang up a morphine drip and titrate it, even.

I used to be very good at this sort of thing.

Back before covid, people still died, you know? And given the specialties my hospital has, we saw more than our fair share of elderly people who'd come in and who definitely were not going out again. I had my spiel down—here's what we're going to do, here's what it's going to look like, here's what you can do as it happens.

All of that was out of the window yesterday, though. I felt like some kind of cave troll emerging into the sunlight, having to interact with strangers face to face.

I wanted to provide them with that Quality Death Experience (tm), and we didn't start off that way, but we got there.

Here's what happens when people die at the hospital, in normal times:

First off, we try to send people home, via hospice, if that's an option. It's almost always better, especially when our visitation rules are still draconian.

After that, we're all about "comfort care."

We kept this patient there because we were going to "compassionately extubate" them, by which we mean pull out their breathing tube, see what happens, and go from there. Oftentimes, patients wouldn't last long enough for hospice to be involved. They'd die pretty quickly, depending on baseline lung function.

At that same time, we turn off any other element of "life support" that's ongoing: any supplemental oxygen, any blood pressure medication, fluids, insulin—we turn all those things off, because the goal's no longer keeping the person alive.

The goal's just to help them die cleanly.

That's what I was having such a hard time explaining yesterday. I mean, I can't just come out and say, "Yeah, the goal here is that they're going die." Except... that's the true-truth, right? I explained all the emphasis on them being "comfortable"—we don't want people to look like they're uncomfortable or air hungry—so in an optimal world, in the best situation in the ICU, it'd just look like your relative was asleep until their heart stopped.

I think a lot of the time, people think about death as a switch, and I may have mentioned that here before; forgive me if I have. The family feels like they've come to this great momentous decision, and they're all ready to yank life away from their relative like a dinner magician with a tablecloth, but no—the actuality of being there is usually much, much slower. It can take days, even. It just is what it is.

The patient got a little rough yesterday—sometimes people drool, and it gives them death rattles, and no one wants to hear that—so you give them medication to dry the spit up and additional sedation to gently decrease their respiratory drive.

And while I'm giving it, one of the relatives in the room with me asks, "So, why don't you just give him a lot of that stuff?"

And I was all, "Well, I don't want to overshoot, you know?"

But of course he doesn't know, nor do you, and neither does anyone else, really.

I said something flippant about killing someone once, because even in the before times I've always been a morbid bitch, and a doctor friend came out of the woodwork to correct me.

"That's not what you're doing. You're just taking them up to the ledge. You're not pushing them over."

What I didn't say then, though, that I couldn't even really conceive of saying until much later, afterwards, after many more times it'd happened, was, "But you're not even on the ledge with me at all! You write the orders and then walk away! You're not there, touching the medications or the patient! Everything's an abstraction for you!!! So how dare you tell me what it feels like to be giving medication that is invariably going to be killing someone, no matter how slowly it happens. Back the eff off."

I may still be angry about this, in my heart.

I thought about explaining the difference between euthanasia and whatever-the-hell-comfort-care-is-supposed-to-be-doing to the family yesterday, but opted not to. They didn't need that, even if it would've felt good for me to get it off my chest.

I did remember one of my old canards: "Just like how babies are born on their own schedules, people die at their own times, too," which seemed to relieve the family some, since it was taking so long.

But that's the goal really. To do this perfect three-point landing, where you get someone to glide, feather-gracefully, out of this world and into the next. Where families have had enough time to say good-bye and hopefully circle around to the story-telling part of things, laughing about memories and sharing photos.

Where it's not about the dying person in there anymore—it becomes about knitting together those who will be left behind.

God, every time I hear someone laughing in a comfort-care room, it's such a burden off of my shoulders—I know I have done my part right.

The last death I had visitors around for was super traumatic for everyone involved, the one where I got the blisters from bagging. So it's been awhile, you know? And that one, like all covid deaths, was just a trainwreck, mostly because it was covid, and it didn't have to happen like that at all.

The only hard part with this one was that our visitation rules are still wonky. My patient was still alive at the end of my shift, and I had their family hidden in there with the curtain. Technically I should've kicked them out hours before. But I'm not an asshole, and if you don't ask questions like "when should they leave?" then no one can get mad at you if they don't. Voila!

I even smuggled up delivery food for them, although I told them it couldn't be a pizza, seeing as we're not allowed to get pizzas anymore, because God forbid we indulge in a potluck now that we've all got our shots.

And then my shift was over, and I handed off the narcotics to the next nurse, who I introduced, and it was me alone in the room with them again.

I felt the need to make some sort of closing statement, because I don't know why, I just did, so I launched off with, "I hope—" and then I paused, and then I just was honest. "I actually don't know what I hope."

Because I didn't—what the fuck do I know, to be hoping? That things go faster, or slower, or for them to be able to hide in there all night?

"I'm just glad you get to be here."

Which was the God's honest truth.

– Cassie

—᷍ᶺ᷍ᶺ᷍—

3/11/20—author newsletter excerpt

Back to real-life updates –

I wound up getting my second vaccine shot in Jan, and boy wasn't that a relief. And then?!?! My ICU actually went through a two-week period at the end of Feb where we didn't have ANY covid patients, which felt like some kind of miracle.

It was too good to last—and I had two of them today—but just that breather... it was so delightful.

And it kind-of proved that a new normal was possible, at the end of all this, and that there will come a time when covid's gone or gone enough. I'll feel the best and safest of all when my husband's able to get his vaccine.

Belatedly, my mom pulled through okay, having had covid—many of you all asked. Sorry to leave you hanging for so long!

I've recently increased my doses of my psych meds, which seem to be helping in general—I think it's fairly evident from newsletters in the past that I'm prone to depression, and working myself to the bone this past winter didn't help anything, obviously, heh. But I am doing better now. I feel like I can see the horizon, now that vaccines are close at hand for those I love, and now that work isn't just all grim-dying all the time.

Here are some recent plant shots for those of you that've made it this far—an echeveria Etna on the left (like the volcano!) and some gorgeous Graptoveria Fred Ives on the right.

More soon when the next new book gets released!

<3

Cassie

3/14/21

I guarantee you there's one patient that's like this, give or take six months of time, in every ICU in America. Mine has two. They're not getting better, nor worse, they're just... there. With lungs too shitty to transfer out. Hanging on, waiting to die.

[CA: this was in response to Kate Garraway's—some famous lady in England—husband having been hospitalized with covid for an entire year. He has apparently been in the ICU the entire time.]

3/14/21—Two Nurses Talking newsletter

Covid-RN-aversary

[CA: I've since realized in doing this book that my actual first date with suspected covid patients was 3/11/20, but since I pinned my "volunteering" tweet on 3/14, I'd assumed that was the date, for the purposes of this newsletter.]

THIS IS CASSIE, and I've prescheduled this post to go live on 3/14, which is the first day I took care of a covid patient at my hospital last year. I know it was 3/14 because I made it my pinned tweet on Twitter, the same Twitter thread I made while walking on my way into work that day.

This is likely going to be a mess of a post, so bear with me.

I'VE ALWAYS HAD a tiny death wish. It's a little echo that follows me around and on an exhausting day whispers, "I wish I was dead," into my ear. Don't worry about me; it's not very loud, and when things are good and I'm well rested and I have things to look forward to, it mostly goes away.

It was louder when I worked on nightshift, just because I was literally tired all the time, but like, look, you've probably heard it too, your very own version.

Is there anyone who's ever driven over an overpass who hasn't thought, "You know, I could yank this wheel over right now"?

The key is to not get stuck there. (I know, because of therapy.) If you keep thinking like that, and it gets louder and sharper, then you need to do something.

The reason I mention this, though, is because it's much the same thought process that made me set my alarm early on 3/14, so I could get into work before the assignment sheets were set in stone—and it's also why I called dibs, on my ICU's private FB group the night before.

My thinking was this: I don't have kids. I don't do elder care. I figured that after so many years of being a burn nurse in isolation gear my game was pretty tight and... basically?

I kind-of wanted to see if I could hack it. And maybe didn't 100% care if I could not.

Nurses at a certain level... aren't exactly built "right." Or, perhaps more honestly, the job molds you into the person it needs you to be, and what it does not need is a normal human being. Normal people aren't interested in hanging out with other people at their lowest moments, possibly covered in shit or blood.

THINGS ARE BETTER NOW than they were last year, for some definitions thereof.

The whole vaccine angle, obviously. AND THE FACT THAT MY ICU JUST WENT TWO WEEKS WITHOUT A COVID PATIENT. (Way to bury the lede, Cassie!)

That was just recently!!! It's over now; we've got them again, but just that brief break—you can't imagine what a difference that made to all of us, to all of our souls, at work.

But if I had known last year, scooping mashed potatoes up off the ground in that one woman's room, that this year would've gone down like this... man, I just don't know.

It's probably a good thing I didn't know how dark it'd get and how long it'd go on for—or how much tragedy and brokenness I'd see, participate in, and feel personally.

It would've been nice to know that there would be a "happy" ending, for me at least, even if not for the half-a-million dead people, victims of our inept government at the time.

. . .

BUT I DON'T KNOW that I'm happy, yet.

I still spent thirty minutes crying like a relative had died last week, over a beloved sickly plant.

I am still—and will always and ever be now—tired of death. My own, I'm not particularly concerned with, but I could go the rest of my life and not need to see anyone else die, ever again, please.

I'm still very mad at people who let me down this past year, and I haven't figured out how to reconcile that with my ongoing life. Should I lance and drain, or should I let it cyst and fester? And to some degree, I know that those aren't even choices I get to consciously make, no matter how much I might want to, you know? Sometimes your psyche just does what it's going to do for you, without your input.

I do know—like everyone else on the planet—that I never want to go through another year like this in my life.

I don't want to scream at a maskless woman in the grocery store as I have a panic attack that, "I SEE PEOPLE DIE ALL THE TIME. WHAT THE FUCK IS WRONG WITH YOU? WHY AREN'T YOU MASKED? WHERE IS YOUR MASK???"

I don't want to shriek at my husband, who's been home alone all day and has come down the stairs to see me as I take off all my clothes after a shift, because he just wants to see another human in real life and say hi, as I shout, "GET BACK! GET BACK! GET BACK!"

I don't want to tell idiots on the internet to stop being selfish dick-weeds and how can they be so cavalier with other people's LIVES, aren't they ashamed of themselves and their actions?

I don't want to have to scream through glass with an n95 on so that my coworkers can hear what it is I need them to bring me, so I don't have to come out of the room I'm in....

Basically, I would like to be done with shouting.

· · ·

SO I HOPE NOW, as things (knocks on wood, crosses fingers, prays to a God she does not believe in) wind down, some sort of protean new normal will arrive.

I don't know what it looks like yet, and to be honest, I haven't started looking very hard.

I'm afraid that the act of accepting that it's time to come out of the cave will somehow set off a new wave of trauma.

ICU nurses and authors have a lot in common, brain-wise, because as a nurse my job is to be the Worst Case Scenario detector, and as an author it's my job to come up with savvy plot twists. That all boils down to the fact that I am smart enough to not be superstitious, while simultaneously actually being superstitious all the time.

I'm like a beat dog, in a manner of speaking, and boy oh boy, did covid beat me down.

But I'm here. Still. Despite not always taking the best care of myself, despite volunteering like a dumbass, despite all the tears, the days I couldn't get out of bed, and the days my alarm went off for work and I had no choice but to go in—

Still.

Here.

I KNOW it's a survivor's prerogative to hype yourself up over having overcome a thing, which isn't fair in the least to all the people who didn't, who likely didn't have a choice, and whose lives had every bit as much meaning to them as yours does to you, possibly more so, depending on their presence or absence of death wishes.

So it'd be bullshit of the highest form to say that I've Learned Things About Myself or that I Can Survive Anything Now, because...have I really? Will I? Could I?

Perhaps more importantly: Would I honestly want to?

The author in me wants to turn this into a story, like I do to most anything else, because stories are sexy and fun and they always have meaning. Beginnings, middles, ends, and "oh wasn't that nice, look at all the friends they made along the way!"

But I think it'd be unfair to pretend that this past year was anything but a shitshow of the highest order, that half a million people died for nothing, and that the psychic scars of that—and of the cognitive dissonance of many more millions of people not caring— aren't going to resonate onward for a very long time.

So I'm not going say anything braggy here about "surviving," because yee-fucking-haw, I met the basic demands of humanity when needed, and part of me even enjoyed it, because I am a person who likes to stare into abysses and run towards spinning knives.

I am very glad the worst of it is over. But I know for a lot of people (and perhaps even for me) there's still more shockwaves to come.

That said, though....

ONE OF THE shitty things about being an author is that you never know when to feel publicly excited about anything.

Most people don't know how book publication works and what a curse it is to bear. You make a sale, but you can't announce it till the publisher does, like six months later, in *Publishers Marketplace*, and by then the joy's seeped out of the moment because your neurotic little brain is already worried about pulling off the sequel. Foreign rights, TV options, etc.—everything's always hush-hush and on someone else's timeframe, and frankly it's exhausting.

So when I was doing traditionally published books I learned to celebrate secretly, with trusted friends, in the moment, because "wins" in the publishing arena are so few and far between.

And so let me tell you this—we've all made it through a year here. I'm absolutely sure all of our pandemic-a-versaries have occurred already or are just about to come up.

I know shit was intolerably sad for so very long. I saw it, and I felt it in my bones. I'm sure some of you have suffered much deeper personal losses than the ones I merely bore witness to, as a bystander.

It's hard to scrape those shadows off of you. I know that too, especially when we're all riding this same trauma-pterosaur together. It's ever so easy for things to echo, and to think we need to diminish any joys we do feel, because we don't want to hurt anyone else along the way.

It's going to be really fucking rocky here for a long time—so maybe I was wrong, and I can guess our new normal—because so many people are so damaged, and it's going to take them so very long to put themselves back together, if they ever even can.

But at the same time—if you're reading this—you're also Still Here.

With me.

And that's worth celebrating, a little. In the moment.

I don't want to gloat, but fuck—we're still alive.

Sometimes it's through no fault of our own and despite our best efforts even, heh.

So yeah. This past year sucked. Hard. Indubitably.

But we've got the rest of this year, above ground, ahead of us now.

And I know it's not always healthy to shut the door on the past—and I'm not asking you to do that, in no way shape or form.

But at least those of us who're still here—we've got a future now.

I was super tempted there to say something grandiose like, "So spend it wisely," because that's a thing a book protagonist's wise mentor would say, heh.

But nah, don't do that! Just be free, get free, do whatever the fuck you want, get laid, get high, just hold onto life now that you're sure you've got one. Figure out what you really want to do and then do it.

I'm not going to dare try to put a positive spin on a year of horrors.

But at the same time, after what we all went through—it wasn't the end of our stories, and it wasn't the end of us. It's OK to be scared and sad about what happened... but if you're moved by any joy right now, as we all stumble out of the darkness together, grasp it with both hands.

Shamelessly.

We're all breathing, my loves, and we've all got more time to go. And personally? I've got more books to write, more overpasses to ignore.

More soon,

– Cassie

3/21/21

Sweet Jesus, you guys!!! Our beloved copyeditor, who did our whole Dragon Called series, went into the hospital with covid on 11/30. I emailed later, two times, and assumed she'd passed, because I knew she was in the ICU. She just EMAILED ME! She just got out on the 13th!!! She's alive!!!

3/23/21

Who has two thumbs and volunteered to work a 16 today, on her first day back after surgery? (They're short five. It was looking grim.)

3/23/21

One of my strongest coworkers: "I can't tell if I've lost my skills, or if I'm just apathetic." Me: "Welcome to nursing in 2021," and then us both sadly cackling.

3/25/21

Oh God, our staffer/vacation approver person is leaving. Between this and new management, I feel like every upper-level person at work I've ever banked points with is gone.

⎯⩗⩘⩗⩘⎯

3/26/21

I find myself dreaming of different, better careers every time I drive into work. Ideally, writing would save me, but I'm becoming increasingly unpicky.

A study finds the United States could've avoided 400,000 deaths and wasting billions of dollars if a mask mandate had been put into place by May 2020. (3/26/21)

3/27/21

Listening to a family member tell a patient that "God is testing their faith" by putting them through this, and, honestly, if that were true, I would pick a different deity.

Heh. I was walking out, masked, to my car in the parking lot and some kids zoomed by on bicycles and pretended to cough really loudly. Not in an antimask way, just in a "kids are assholes" way.

Little do they know I've just been inoculating in covid for 12 hours.

3/27/21

YEAR OF THE NURSE   303

Here's a rundown of three different conversations I got to have with different people today, which all were the same thing, just in different ways. (Warning, sad shit incoming.)

With cops: "Hey. Yeah. No, they're alive. Yeah, we thought they were going to die, too."

"No, they're not gonna be the same."

"Yeah, they were 'lucky.'"

"No, they're not brain dead. That's its own weird medical thing, this isn't that."

"Where are they going to be in 30 days? Probably in a skilled nursing facility." (I guess the cops have a "fatality" window on certain things, for their paperwork, and if you die outside the window it doesn't count.)

"No, no one is pulling the plug."

"No, nothing is likely to change."

Conversation 2: "So we can't just turn off the sedation to see if they wake up. They're having neuro-issues, and that would hurt them."

"I saw their MRI, and I know neuro talked to you. I wish I could tell you differently, but I can't."

"In my experience, someone with injuries like this doesn't get better, but there's always a chance. I'm not God."

"I know you want the meds off, but that's not safe."

"It's a brain injury. We have to do what's safest for the patient. These things take time to heal—if they're going to heal. And I can't predict the future. I so, so, so wish I could."

"We just have to wait it out right now and give them the safest chance we can."

"I can't make any promises. I'm very sorry."

Conversation 3: "I know you want a miracle. But this is a brain stem injury and we're pretty far out from when it happened. This is likely the functionality they're going to be at for the rest of their life."

"Yes, they'll continue to absorb the blood, but the initial pressure damage the blood did, pressing their brains inside their skull—that tissue damage is very likely permanent."

"Of course you can keep praying."

"I know. My heart breaks for you."

Okay, that's off my chest. Back to the book mines.

3/30/21

The longer I write, the more I begin to believe that everyone has just one story to tell, but if you're lucky and try for long enough, you can write it with more eloquence and at higher volume.

3/30/21

I've been thinking—shh, I've already written 3k today, I'm allowed to wander—and I think you shouldn't be able to opt out of a covid vaccine until you've seen five people die of covid at a hospital. Like up close and personal. Their last 72 hrs. times five.

3/31/21

All that is in me wants to call in sick tomorrow to write. Can't do it, though. Just got to shove two more days of my life thru the meatgrinder and then a weekend off. How bad can it be? ... uhhhh. Well, we'll find out.

APRIL 2021

4/1/21

Perhaps other people need to hear this as well, so chances are if you ever think, "Huh, maybe I should up my psych meds, under my Dr.'s supervision," you're right.

(That was written by someone who really should've done this 6 months ago, but better late than never.)

4/2/21

Our covid numbers at work are creeping up slightly. I have a great assignment, though, but all I want to do is go home and write.

No breaks today. Not enough staff.

4/4/21

Work's been short this whole past week. We're not overrun with covid anymore; we're overrun with apathy.

Everyone has PTO to burn from "pitching in" all last year, staff is burnt, and our new management isn't allowed to incentivize us, so all these texts and calls go unread.

4/7/21

There's a palpable sense of relief in taking care of covid patients, now that my husband's been vaccinated.

It feels that much more manageable.

4/7/2021—password protected journal

My besties realized we'd all be vaccinated in time for a husband's 50th in May, over a weekend I'd already gotten plane tickets out to see some relatives.

God bless Southwest, because I have never changed a flight so fast. There was no way I'm missing the first party with my besties in a year.

We're going to spend the weekend in Santa Cruz, my husband's going shooting with all the boys, and I am going to get drunk and snuggle with all of my friends. Can't wait!

4/7/21

Our new management seems to not care if we ever get breaks again.

Spending the end of my 17-hr. shift here at work, sustained by soda, sparkling water, and the @AnniesAnnuals spring flower catalog.

4/8/21

Already locked in for another 16-hr. shift. Going to pay for my upcoming new fancy rowing machine outright.

4/8/21

I just walked into an unexpectedly high monitor on one of our mobile computers and skinned off a piece of my forehead.

I would like to go home now.

4/10/21

I went into an empty patient room singing "Total Eclipse of the Heart," and got startled when a visitor came out of the bathroom. Super glad they missed me singing "Special K" by Placebo earlier, as I hung ketamine.

4/11/21

I'm not working extra today. Someone high five me.

4/12/21

I had very few fucks to spend before the pandemic, and I will have even fewer after.

4/13/21

My dad, who had asymptomatic covid in Dec [CA: my stepdad, who I call my dad, had it at the same time as my mom, apparently], just had a stroke this morning. They caught it fast and gave him tPA, but I feel in my heart of hearts that (it being an ischemic stroke) it was covid related.

4/13/21

After having worked in an ICU this past year, I would literally get any vaccine on the market shoved into my arm, while I, and possibly the person providing it, were blindfolded, even if I knew it was mixed with lead & arsenic, which I know they aren't.

Like they could spin the wheel of goddamned theoretical contaminants, and I'd be all, "You know, guinea worms don't sound so bad, by comparison. Shoot one of those fuckers in there too."

We've left the people of Flint, MI waiting this whole effing time to get their pipes cleaned up, you drink water out of plastic bottles in neon colors all day, you think Starbucks is healthy, and everyone likes to feed their livers wine.

Unless you, you anti-vax MFer, are sitting at home, encased in pure cotton that you harvested your damn self, breathing air that you personally pumped through a HEPA filter, and eating food that you harvested out of your own effing garden... get your fucking vaccine.

4/14/21

Ativan doesn't solve all the problems, but it does downshift them quite nicely.

4/15/21

Y'all, my folks and my brother are both first-shot vaccinated now, and I wasn't 100% sure that was going to happen.

You know that cheesy fictional "breath you didn't know you were holding"? It is indeed a real thing.

4/15/21

Trying to stay vigilant about recognizing my PTSD-hypervigilance is going swimmingly, lolsob.

4/15/21

I should probably get to bed before my nearly inevitable 16-hr. shift tomorrow. (Is it a good idea? No. Am I going do it anyways if I can? Yes, because I ain't never met scissors I didn't want to run with. Plus, I have Sat off to recoup, *shrug*.)

4/16/21

Everyone I know who works in a hospital is burnt out to within an inch of their lives.

My friend was excited that, when she had a patient go comfort care the other day, she still managed to feel something.

People still want the best from us, and actually they still deserve the best from us, but there is just no fucking room at the inn. The barrel is empty. One and all.

And we're running out of supplies because the person who usually ordered supplies for us is gone. So that is amazing. And our union is sending us emails asking how much of a strike we can afford this summer.

I know that it's not a good idea for me to be working under these conditions. But at the same time, it's not like me not working is going to fix anything? It's not like there's a bunch of bright-eyed and bushy-tailed ICU baby nurses waiting in the wings.

I'm leaving work tonight with one of my friends who is equally burnt out, and we realize, in the lobby of our floor as a guy tries to get out on the wrong floor, that he is actually a patient going AWOL.

He's all casual about it of course. But he asks directions to a church, and we tell him he needs to go down to the first floor, and we see that he's wearing an ID band.

We don't get into his elevator with him because he looks scruffy.

But we're both going to the same place, so she and I debate in our elevator on whether we're actually going to be good people when we get to the first floor and help him out by having security escort him back to his room.

We do it, mind you. She distracts him and while I go get security. But like, the talk was real.

I don't know what to do with any of that. And I doubt you do, either. I guess thanks for listening and we'll see how tomorrow goes when we get there.

***

I THINK that moment in the elevator with my coworker was probably my inflection point.

We were both in that elevator, legitimately hoping that someone else would deal with the patient trying to escape. Or that we could both just simultaneously look the other way.

It was almost eight PM and we were exhausted by then, by that day, that month, that whole fucking year.

We both decided to do the right thing... but the conversation we had about *not* doing it was real.

And honestly, if I'd been in the elevator alone, it might've been a coin toss.

Do you know how hard it is to be a good person?

Relentlessly?

It's exhausting.

I get so tired of caring sometimes, when no one else does. I mean, I know it's my job and my ethos... but what do you do when there's nothing left inside?

And the flip side of doing the right thing is that, so often, even when you try, no one takes your advice.

Coming home that day, I found my husband outside, taking in our neighbor's garbage cans, because she felt too weak.

She had a wet cough, and I knew she'd been vaccinated and she swore she hadn't seen anyone. I was pretty sure she had congestive heart failure—if she didn't have an infection, the reason her cough was "wet" was because fluid was accumulating in her lungs.

Your heart has two jobs—it pumps deoxygenated blood into your lungs, and then once that blood's become oxygenated, it pumps it back out through your body to feed your cells, like we've talked about before.

If your heart becomes incompetent for some reason, because some of the vessels out of your heart are blocked and not enough blood moves forward, some of that blood will back up into your lungs, giving you a wet cough, as your heart becomes "congested" with blood and experiences a type of "heart failure" in that it's no longer properly doing its job.

I figured this was what was happening to her.

I tried to talk her into letting me take her to the hospital. She said I must be "missing work," and teased that I was scaring her, though we both knew it was true.

My husband, who had no interest in going to the hospital with her (although he is a good person)—could tell my pressing her was making her a little upset. So he gave her an out, saying, "Well, your friend's coming over tomorrow, right? So you can see how you feel, then."

And she was all, "Oh, yes, tomorrow!"

And I was all, *here we go again.*

I try to tell people to do the right thing.

But so often, people just don't want to listen.

I whispered to my husband on our way back to our front door what was most likely happening to her, and he freaked out that he'd "killed" her by giving her an "out," but honestly, she really didn't want to go in—I did try very hard to convince her. I didn't precisely want to take an 80-plus-year-old person into the hospital, emergency-style, in the dregs of a pandemic, either. I mean, what if she picked up something worse there?

Should I have made my case more forcefully? I don't want to be an asshole, and I always want to give people some autonomy, so I sucked up not being listened to, again.

Cassie's not my real name. You might have picked that up. (I don't super hide my real name, but I'm also not Elena Ferrante.)

I chose Cassie back when I became an author because I always have to wear a badge at work, and I didn't really want my patients Googling me. Especially at my old hospital. While I loved it, we had a lot of sketchy patients there. My thinking at the time was that they deserved to know that they weren't getting put into a book—and I'd never met a Cassie I didn't like..

If I had known how often being a Cassie in 2020 would feel like being Cassandra of Troy, though, cursed to speak the truth but no one ever listening... I might have picked differently.

And sure enough, when my neighbor's friend came in to check on her the next day, they took her to the hospital, where she got two stents placed.

———————————————————

4/16/21

Gorges on burrata, Doritos, and moody music till I can't stand myself anymore. I don't want to have any feelings other than a stomachache and some guy's piano solo.

4/17/21

Decided to go into work tomorrow. Just got to put two days in, then five days off—this is my year of using PTO. I put in for it awhile back.

I can do anything for 48 hrs.

4/18/21

My patient at work today didn't take the vaccine when it was first offered to him, for "Resident Evil" reasons.

I wasn't aware we lived in Raccoon City, but apparently.

[CA: Resident Evil is a popular video game franchise with a zombie-contagion virus.]

4/18/21

In hindsight, this 16 was a bad idea.

If you want your loved ones to die at home in peace, please involve hospice instead of waiting a week and then doing a full court press.

4/22/21

I've now managed to go to sleep for three nights without Ambien, setting a recent-me record.

4/22/21

So what do people who aren't perpetually anxious do with their whole day?

Three in 10 healthcare workers have considered leaving their profession. Over half are burnt out. Six in 10 say stress from the pandemic has harmed their mental health. (4/22/21)

4/24/21

I would like to not be an ICU nurse anymore.

I don't precisely know how to escape it yet, where I'll go, or what I'll do, but the first step is admitting it out loud.

4/25/21

I'm turning off Twitter off on my phone for a bit so I don't say anything stupid.

My mental health isn't super great, and since I'm prone to oversharing, this is safest.

Be back in a week or two.

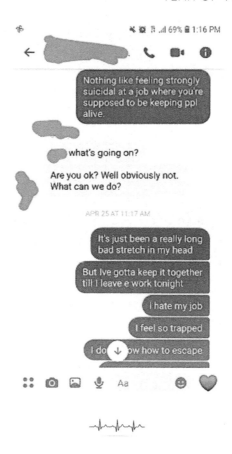

THERE WAS NO REAL one thing that triggered me texting my friends or how I felt that day.

It was just the accumulation of a thousand tiny sorrows. For months upon months, any time we were scared, anytime we wanted to cry, anytime we wanted to hug each other, anytime we wanted to shake a family and say, "Why are you making us torture this person?", me and every other nurse in America just had to shove it down.

Shove it down, shove it down, shove it down. It might as well have been a mantra.

I've come to realize that all of the memories I've put into boxes—they're not the memories themselves anymore. They've just composted into tears.

And all the tears I couldn't cry last year, and possibly for years beforehand, there was just no more room for them inside me.

I started crying and I couldn't stop.

I cried through my first break and then again through my second, just sitting quietly at the back of the still-empty waiting room, tears streaming down my cheeks until they were hidden by my mask.

I really did think, like an idiot, that I could tough things out, but we were downgrading one of my patients and there were no admits on the horizon. A coworker with greater seniority asked to go home, but I caught my charge nurse and said, "No. I am having a mental health crisis. It needs to be me," and she came into the utility room with me so I could cry some on her.

By then my friends had contacted my husband, who had messaged me, threatening to call 911 if I didn't message him. Luckily, I looked at my phone—I keep the volume off during work hours—and messaged him back, right before my opportunity to leave early occurred.

Then I cried all the way down the hall. I cried in the breakroom, got a very solid hug from a coworker, and then cried all the way out to my car.

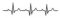

4/25/21—password protected journal

Today was a bottom-of-the-barrel kind of day.

Suicidal stuff incoming, not going to hide it, so just be aware.

I think the whole psychic burden of all last year is coming due in a big way. And I just couldn't handle it at work today. I told my girls-chat that it was ironic that I was trying to keep people alive when all I really wanted to do was die, and they went into Cassie-protection-overdrive.

I didn't want to bother my husband, because you know, when you're in the depths, you make bad decisions, and he's been stressed lately himself, so I thought I could keep my shit together till I came home.

But some of my friends reached out to him and he reached out to me to yell with love, and I hid in an equipment supply room and cried with my charge nurse for five minutes, and they figured out a way for me to get to go home, staffing-wise. Luckily we were even downgrading one of my patients, which made it easy.

I don't like being weak, as you might imagine. I like to think of myself as an impervious object, who has seen the worst, and in some cases done the worst to other people, seeing as being a burn nurse was oftentimes being a congenial professional torturer. Vast swaths of my body are covered with tattoos, once upon a time I had 17 piercings, I used to do martial arts, I still torture myself exercise-wise regularly as a form of control, and so it is so, so, so bizarre to me that there is a piece of me that is so delicate and fragile that all it wants to do some-days is fly away, out the nearest window.

I remember when we were in the thick of covid, trying to save so many people whom we knew were dying, and thinking, "Man, if any of those people were me, I would just tell you to stop. Like... I am not worth all that effort. Truly."

And... I'm not scared of death? Pain, eh, depends, but death? What is there to be afraid of? I don't really count. In a hundred years no one will know who I was. In the scheme of things, we're all galactically insignificant, so it would be stupid for me to fear my own non-existence. Heaven doesn't exist and neither does hell, so, sure, while life is a celebration, of some sort yet to be determined, I'll hang out here with my husband and the cats, but you can bet money now that at the end of my useful existence I will choose how to go and I will go —into the West, into the Dark—whatever, with a minimum of fighting.

Right now it's just this twofold thing, where I really don't like my job anymore. We're undersupported, usually understaffed, we're running out of supplies because I don't even know the fuck why but it's embarrassing, and morale there is at an all-time low.

And then writing stuff is just meh.

I've written 32 books in my 45 years on this planet and still haven't managed to assemble anything even vaguely career-like out of them. No one could tell you what a Cassie Alexander story was if they tried, I don't think.

I just keep trying and trying, really hard, with all my might, and getting hurt. Over and over and over.

And it sucks, you know? Because like... I'm really fucking good.

It would hurt less if I knew I still needed to get better—like for my nine books that didn't sell pre-*Nightshifted*, I knew my skills were leveling up.

But now, I'm pretty fucking badass and that still doesn't mean— nor guarantee—a goddamned thing.

And I know writing's not, nor has ever been, a meritocracy. But, Jesus, really? Do I have to work this fucking hard? Have I earned no easy-breaks through virtue of karma alone? How many lives does a bitch have to save, I mean really?

And I see people—obviously only small portions of their lives online, I know, I know, but still—who have all this copious, magical free time, writing more than me, getting more opportunities than I have, tie-ins, comic books, TV-deals, expounding cogently on multiple media-related topics. Like, I don't think I could tell you the plot of a single MCU movie if I tried, while here I am really just trying to get by and stay mediocrely relevant. (Hooray, being a covid-nurse made that facet of my life popular. Hooray, everyone's going to go back to being normal and never think of me again, because why would you want to play with the broken doll in the corner when you could play with whatever's today's new model is?)

I am very, deeply, anxious about everyone else going back to normal and me just... not. Me, being trapped here in the behind lands, with all these feelings no one wants to feel anymore or think about, pain no one wants to see in their Shiny New Futures. I have a very, very, very strong sympathy for Vietnam Vets now.

Anyhow.

I've reached out to my old therapist, asking for an emergency appointment. I've taken the next two days off of work. I've emailed my endocrinologist in case this is some lovely "your thyroid hates you again"-type thing. I've deleted Twitter from my phone, so I won't be tempted to post shit like this over there, without context. And I've let the moderators here know they're on their own and I'll abide by whatever they decide here for the next two weeks.

More Ativan in the interim, I suppose. Hell, I even took a vitamin in case it helps.

Your shambling derelict,

Cassie

THUS BEGIN my attempts to find a therapist that my health insurance covers. I began with their employee-assistance program—I call the number, and the nice lady asks me what's wrong with me, and I say, "I think I have PTSD," and immediately begin crying.

She seems sympathetic, takes my information, and promises to get back in touch.

I'm freaking out a little bit now because I know I cannot go back into work the next two days that I'm supposed to be on.

I have been "crazy" before, and might be crazy again, but that period there was the worst of it.

I usually use the metric 'Would I want me to be my nurse?' And if the answer's yes, then I go in, and if the answer's no, I call in sick.

The problem with last year, though, was that there was literally no one else to pick up slack, ever. We were short almost all the time—at least when shit got real.

That made it hard to allow myself those moments.

I moderate a large password-protected board for writers, which is where some of these entries are harvested, and a week before all this went down, someone had done something asshattish on there, and I kinda-sorta did something asshattish back to them. They flounced off and I was genuinely upset.

Then it occurred to me, "Oh, my dad has had a stroke. Oh, I wrote down here that I was taking an Ativan. Perhaps that was not the day that I should've been making solo moderation decisions."

But at the time, and through the lens of what I'd been through—I thought I could hack it, because why not?

I went to work when my mother had covid, for christsake.

―᚜ᚋᚌᚋ᚜―

I SPENT a lot of last year rowing to the TV show *Hannibal*, because I am goth through and through, and something the very messed up main character said midway through really resonated with me: "I may be broken, but I'm the only one you've got."

I stopped rowing right at that very moment and stared at the screen, truly feeling seen for the first time since covid had begun.

―᚜ᚋᚌᚋ᚜―

I—AND literally millions of other nurses—went through last year feeling entirely unvalued and endangered. We were forced to participate in a quantity of death and horror that most of you will never comprehend, by people for whom mandating said deaths was only a theoretical abstraction—and who apparently gave no shits if that level of murder went on and on, with no end in sight.

It broke me.

It broke us.

And yet we were the only ones you've got.

WE HAD no choice but to keep it together, then. For our patients, our coworkers, and ourselves.

To have had any introspection at the time was the same as practically signing a suicide note.

NOW, though... oh, now....

4/26/21

Since I didn't flounce off of Twitter, it's OK if I come back early now that I'm sane...er. I still haven't reinstalled it on my phone, though.

If my bosses give me shit about taking three days off without a sick note, I'm going to show them my foiled attempts to get a therapist.

I am a person of means, with health insurance and money, and if it is this hard for me to find someone, me who has all the support in the world, what the hell chance do other people have, who've probably been brain-hurt longer than me, besides?

Luckily, my old therapist can get me in on Weds evening, after her dentist appt. I'm just going be in standby mode after 6 pm, waiting, and I can afford to pay out of pocket.

I was going through old story ideas the other day, combing thru them for something to write that might give me energy, and one of them was a lit RPG about someone's attempts to get mental health access, and that hits a little close to home.

Tucker Carlson tells people to harass people who wear face masks outside, saying that "masks are just a sign of obedience" and if you see children in masks you should call CPS because that is abuse. (4/26/21)

─╴╴╴╴╴╴╴╴╴

HAVE you ever had someone voting Republican back down on a point?

I have, but just the once.

WHEN THE SENATE was going to repeal the Affordable Care Act yet again—you might remember John McCain's stunning swing vote saving it—I went up to see my folks to try to put a human face on things.

I kept thinking that these, the people that raised me to be good and kind, to perhaps too literally read the Bible and try to do all that stuff like Jesus does, if they could only understand what it was like to need healthcare in American society, surely they would change their minds.

And so, I talked to my dad about stuff, because I look up to him and I feel like if I just try hard enough, I'll flip the switch to make him see. I explain to him that if this law passes, that every single burn patient I have ever had will have a pre-existing condition—and I point out to them that I, also, have a pre-existing heart condition—and that we're all going to be sunk, healthcare-wise, if this happens.

I also cried, then.

And, while it worked, while my dad told my mom to tell me that he'd changed his mind about it, prior to McCain voting, I think I did myself a disservice.

You see, I spent a lot of Trump's presidency, and the run up to it, trying to change their minds by relating policies I knew he'd enact to me personally, in an effort to put a human face on things, rather than whatever the hell Fox was selling them that week.

That led to a particularly fraught Thanksgiving as I confessed to my ex-husband's grey rape of me, comparing it to Trump's well-documented history of sexual abuse, and me nearly fainting.

I know, you've read this whole book so far and you likely think me highly emotional, but please trust that I am not a fainter. I have seen flesh burned black to bone, I have seen leaking brains, I have seen blood in a volume that would make most despair, and yet there I was, the world going dark, my arm draped around my dad's neck as everything narrowed in.

Grey rape, for those not familiar with the term, is kind of in the category of "sex that you think you can push through because you feel like you have no choice, and maybe you're not shouting 'no' at the time, due to whatever elements got you into that position in the first place." You might not have a legal leg to stand on later, and you may not even realize it's occurring at the time, because of the coercive element when it is happening, but it can still fuck you up, just like any violation of your personal autonomy.

I feel like, though, in these attempts to make the abstract personal, I merely lacquered on an accumulation of over-dramatic crazy in their eyes, which probably made it easier to ignore me later, like when I called my mother up, hoping that she'd be sympathetic to the fact that I was in danger at work when we were low on gowns.

It was probably easier and felt safer for her to believe that I was exaggerating at the time, than it was to acknowledge that by the act of voting for Republican policies, and continuing to support their aims, she had had any personal hand in my plight.

I remember crying in my car when Trump won, and calling my mother, and her admitting that they'd voted for him, and me howling, "How could you?" because I knew, as someone working in healthcare and married to a lawyer who works at non-profits trying to protect access to the internet, that we were about to get significantly boned.

They'd just gone and put my personal and financial future at risk and for what, an orange clown?

So.

Have you heard of the Paradox of Tolerance?

Even if you're not familiar with it personally, you've likely experienced it before. Let me explain....

Basically, it states that if you're in a place—online or real-life, socially—that operates sheerly on "tolerance!" then everything there winds up in a fascist-Nazi cesspool.

Because if you revere "tolerance!" above all else, eventually intolerant people will use your "tolerance!" against you and drive everyone else out.

Thus, in order to create a truly safe space for people to exist, you need to be intolerant of intolerance, rather than merely tolerant of everything and hoping for free-market-goodwill to do the rest.

MY RELATIONSHIP with my ex-husband wasn't great for many reasons, but chief among them was this: the man could not apologize. I do not think the words "I'm sorry," ever left his mouth. It was just not a thing, for whatever reason, that he was capable of.

But in real life, in jostling up against other human beings on a day-to-day basis, there is a certain amount of apology required, to grease the wheels of society, as it were, even if you don't even fully mean it. When someone says they've had a bad day, when someone's stubbed their toe, when someone files taxes late, a sympathetic, "I'm sorry" is in order. It shows that you're listening to the other person, taking their complaints seriously, and that you are on their side.

If one person in a relationship never says, "I'm sorry," then the burden of that falls on the other person in the relationship, to not only say their portion of the apologies, but also to take on their partner's missing half.

I FEEL like we're experiencing the Paradox of Tolerance now, writ large politically, in that the Left is barely waking up to the need to aggressively deplatform liars—i.e., to be intolerant of intolerance—and we're also realizing that the Right will never, ever, apologize or say, "I'm sorry," which is its own kind of trauma.

None of those people who voted for Trump really care that now, as of yesterday (6/3/21), six hundred thousand people have died of covid.

I don't think that even one of them has looked back at their actions this past year with shame or regret—because if they had, why the hell would they have voted for more of him?

AND SO THE rest of us, the rational people who don't want other humans to die needlessly, are left dragging them along like a millstone around our necks, this sociopathic contingent of society that has no political agenda other than to be verbally jerked off by hate from Carlson's ilk because it makes them feel good.

HOW ARE WE, the sane ones, to take this? Knowing that people around us would gladly chum the waters with our countrymen for sport?

4/27/21

A dove is nesting in a succulent pot outside. It's her deck now.

4/27/21—password protected journal

Thanks for all the love, y'all, and to people who've emailed/texted me, etc.

Yesterday was a pretty flat day. Sat in bed for a long time. Sat on the couch for a long time. Just kind of not doing much or thinking much.

I finally forced myself to go outside and lay down ant bait. Ants are all over my succulent flowerstalks, trying to have an aphid party, the bastards. The doorbell rang. I know because it makes a horrible BLAT sound downstairs.

It goes off once, and I'm all, in my head, "I'm fucking crazy today. My husband needs to deal with that," and then it goes off again, and I'm all, "goddammit, man, get the door,'" and then a minute later he's shouting outside for me to come up, and one of my Santa Cruz friends drove up to surprise me with cake and booze.

We hung out for a while and that was nice.

I tried to get my hospital system to set me up with a shrink. They found me one who was approximately a billion years old and only available Fri/Sat, so I wouldn't be able to see them till 5/29th. I asked them to find me a new-new one, and I haven't heard back yet.

Today I also Attempted Errands.

I went to exercise, because if I'm going to feel bad, I might as well feel bad having exercised, and it was so nice and sunny out, and then I was all, "maybe I'm an asshole who called in sick for nothing,'" because it felt like my shit was together for a brief moment, and then a song I liked came on my playlist and I was sobbing in the car.

Then I went to try to go get my thyroid labs drawn, but I didn't realize the way my Dr. ordered them meant I had to go to my hospital system—Why is everything not electronic? Why?—so I had waited for 45 mins for nothing and then started crying on the poor lady there, who had to explain to me how labs work.

After that, I got to go see a friend who was in Alameda today, and I cried some more there, and then we talked for a few hours and that was good—I came home exhausted and took a nap.

I've got another friend coming up from Santa Cruz tomorrow for a walk around the lake, and my old therapist has fit me in tomorrow at noon, so that's good.

I'm nervous about explaining my absences at work, seeing as I've technically been gone 2.5 days, and you need a Dr.'s note for over three days, but seeing as we don't currently have a staffer and my interim manager is leaving next Friday I'm probably okay, heh.

I'm more nervous about going to Texas on Thurs, which is probably a vastly bad idea on my part. I would cancel but my dad did just have a stroke, and if it happened again and went poorly and I didn't see him because of my broke-brain, I would whip myself about it until the end of time.

It may be good? Maybe being with family will be good for me? (hahahahaha.) I'm worried enough about my work thinking I'm crazy now; at least my family already thinks I'm crazy, *shrug emoji*, so hey. If someone says something dumb about masks or covid I will probably either start bawling or shouting in an unhinged fashion; hooray. If shit gets really bad, I'm flying Southwest, so it'll be easy to make flight changes and I can get out of dodge quickly.

This is the longest I've felt like this ever, I think. I have an appt with my psychiatrist the day after I get back, so we can talk then about me getting some Klonopin. I don't think I actually need it, so much as I need to know that I have it. Usually, by the time I ask for a med, the time for that med has long come and gone. It's sort of the process of realizing that I need it that means things are changing. Here's to hoping.

What sucks is that she's new to me, and I've only seen her for one visit before. My old doctor left that practice, *sigh*, so I don't know if she'll believe me?

I also don't know if I'll have my act together enough to work next week, post-Texas. I don't know how to fully get out of working, either, like, who I need a note from or anything. I don't particularly want to go to suicide summer camp, as a friend called her outpatient psych treatment. Like, I shouldn't have to make myself inpatient to get notes from people? Because ugh. I'm mildly functional, sheesh. I just need some time.

Apparently FMLA is an option, if I can get the right documentation. I don't know how to do that yet, but hopefully my trusty old therapist, who I will be paying out of pocket for tomorrow, knows how to work things. I'll call my health insurance's person again tomorrow, too, for a hopefully cheaper therapist hook-up. I get a whopping ten sessions a calendar year, and it's almost May, so I'd better get cracking, heh.

That's that. Yeehaw.

4/28/21

Y'all, my beloved old therapist is helping me to get FMLA. I really get some time off. For the first time in three days, I want to cry for a good reason, heh.

4/28/21—password protected journal

The bad news: My old therapist's out-of-pocket rates have doubled.

The good news: She is TOTALLY ON BOARD WITH FMLA.

I just got off the phone with my work's HR dept, and assuming they don't bone me somehow, I'll be off through 6/6.

Holy shit, what a miracle that would be.

My old therapist was all, "Yeah, I was wondering how you were doing and I was surprised I hadn't heard from you...." The last time we talked was back last March, when I was dealing with my own goddamned brother sending me anti-mask memes, heh, and I couldn't hack it anymore.

When I look back at all the shit I've had to deal with this year, between "don't live your life in fear" bullshit family stuff, and reality stuff—my mom getting covid against literally all of my advice and best efforts—and the sheer volume of depressing hospital stuff, talking to family members via facetime at work as people died, the Hellraiser "such sights to show you" shit I've seen, keeping people alive way past their expiration dates because families didn't get it, or watching people die who didn't have to if other people could've just skipped Christmas for once, just on and on and on.... I totally emotion-barfed on her, which I'd feel bad about, but it's her job, and like, in context, giving her the very high-level run down of this whole past year of moral distress and cognitive dissonance, in addition to my pre-existing underlying depression and anxiety... like whyyyyyyyyy the fuck did I ever think I could manage this all on my own?

It was the first time I've ever tried to explain to another person what A Year Of Being Me During the Pandemic has been, fully, without making light of something, downplaying something else, being sarcastic, ironic, or trying to make myself sound gruff and macho.

I guess up until now I had no choice, really, to do all that, to cope. But shit, no wonder I lost it.

I'm still trying to find cheaper care access through my health insurance, but I will gladly pay out of pocket for essentially a month-long sick note.

The nice thing about talking to her, too, is that I feel comfortable really telling her how I feel because I know she's not going to commit me, heh. Starting off a new therapy relationship with, "hey, work's made me suicidal" didn't seem like it was going to be super profitable right off the bat, as true as it may be. My poor husband, he truly loves me, and he was really worried about having to Do Something on Sunday. I'm glad we dodged that. I hope I can rest enough that him having to Do Something doesn't happen.

I'm still astounded, although I shouldn't be, that the only way for me to have accessed emergency mental health care in a timely fashion through my insurance would've been to call 911 or go in and commit myself. That's fucking scary.

I'm so lucky I have my old therapist still and can afford to take a month off with no pay.

Just wow.

I know, knowing me, that I'll stress out about going back at the end of this... but that's a problem for much more well-rested June-Cassie to deal with.

For right now, May-Cassie has a whole goddamned month off.

YOU MAY HAVE REALIZED I've glissandoed over me actually feeling suicidal and moved on.

There's a lot of reasons for that.

Part of me is worried I can't be true to that moment, the way it felt at the time, more so than I already was in my contemporaneous journaling.

And part of me is worried that to think a lot about how that feels is to invoke it, like summoning a shitty demon.

I have friends, good and true, my husband is wonderful, and I know there's light and life in the world, and excellent cats but....

There's some quality of feeling like that—it's like being at the bottom of a well, trapped hip deep in cool, slick mud. And everyone you know and love is up at the top of the well, on the surface, shouting their feelings down, trying to tell you how much you mean to them and how they want you to stick around, but the more they yell the deeper the well gets. Things echo inside of it, becoming distorted. Vehement tones dampen.

Let me tell you this: at least in my case, when I am in the well—it isn't that I disbelieve you. If you tell me I am awesome, or cool, or you like me very much—I believe that you feel like that about me. Completely.

It's just that I feel like it doesn't matter.

And I think that's more a me-failing, than a you-failing, really.

Because I suffer from the compulsion of wanting to matter. I mean, shit, it's why I've been writing my whole life, isn't it? To change lives and minds? And why I go to work, and volunteer to do the hardest jobs—not to seem heroic, but because something inside of me desperately wants my life to fucking count.

So when I sieve my hands through the remnants of last year and all the memories run through my fingers and there's nothing there to hold—that's what gets me, I think.

None of it had to happen.

None of it mattered.

Not those deaths, not that pain, and not my life as I lived it, besides.

And when the vast quantities of things I had done that didn't matter seemed to outweigh the things I had managed to accomplish, there seemed no point in trying any more.

EMPIRICALLY, I know that that is not true. Especially now, when I'm sitting in a bucket, oh, three-fourths of the way out of the well. My loved ones' words have become clearer and I am more ready to hear them.

But it's just hard to want to keep climbing up the rope, because up there, everything still hurts. Up there, I have to keep trying to make people change. And I'll keep having to go to work and try to save people again.

Just knowing in a theoretical sense that I matter is not enough. I need to be able to push through that and buffer some strength for later—I need to find that mythical thing called "resilience!" that so many of our emails from management want to sell us on.

You know what creates resilience?

Being adequately compensated for the danger you were put in and the trauma you've seen. Feeling listened to at the highest levels of society and government. Knowing that the shit you have gone through is not, absolutely not, going to happen ever again. Knowing that people are going to shut down anti-vaxers and covid-deniers the second they open up their idiot mouths. Knowing that people who care about your health and wellbeing are in charge, and that they'll protect you and your patients when you are at work again.

That would be a start.

You know what doesn't create resilience?

A one-hour continuing education credit paid for out of my own goddamned educational leave.

. . .

NURSES IN FRANCE got a raise last summer and if they died fighting covid their families became "wards of the state," were given material support, and their children future scholarships.

As of 5/5/21, 3600 healthcare workers have died of covid in the US—that's 1.2 September 11ths, for people keeping score. Every single time the government—Bernie, Harris, Biden—discussed giving additional pay to healthcare workers, four million-plus people held their breath, hoping that This Time We Might Really Be Recognized.

And not fucking once did any of them come through.

I'm going to keep voting for people like them because I clearly don't like the alternative. But I won't lie, having been forced to rise to a once-in-a-lifetime occasion, and carrying the psychic scars forward with me now—being ignored, and knowing that no one gives a shit about the ones of us in the line of fire who did die, that burns.

MAY 2021

5/1/21

Man, if this past year didn't put you on benzos, I hate you or I'm sad that you don't have access to mental healthcare.*

    * Wild generalization for humorous intent. As a lady on the internet, I have to use disclaimers, lest I attract pedants.

    (P.S. I likely don't hate you.)

5/1/21

Well, if you had told me a few months ago that my first restaurant experience in 15 months was going to be at a Benihana in Frisco, TX, I would have laughed.

5/1/21

Is everyone just going to pretend that none of this ever happened?

I do see the value in moving forward, when you can, but...
are there other people like me, for whom that's going to take a
while?

Or am I going to get left behind?

Because out at dinner tonight.... I felt so left behind, you all
have no idea. My brother made fun of me for wearing a mask,
and I had to go into the bathroom and have a panic attack.

I came back out and told him I'd watched people die for a
year. He said he didn't want to hear it.

And then I sat down and we tried to finish having a
normal dinner out in public like normal people.

I feel so fucked.

Should I have fought harder? Yelled more? Brought up that
he and his wife had gotten their second shots literally yesterday?

I wish my panic didn't short circuit my "fight for myself"
brain.

I wish I weren't always the odd man out in my family.

I wish someone else had my back.

I didn't tell them anything about my mental health crisis
this past weekend, nor my month of FMLA coming up.

Because then they'd just think I'm weaker and crazier
than they already do.

Somehow I went through 2020 as a covid nurse, and yet
they think I'm still the weak one.

In hindsight, having my first dinner at a restaurant indoors, in
public, in Texas, after fifteen months, was a vastly bad idea.

We had reservations for 3:45 pm. I assumed that we were going
to be the first dinner seating, and that the restaurant would be empty.
And I did want to go out and have fun with my family, right?

Because I don't enjoy being the black sheep.

I love them.

I crave their love and acceptance like a small yappy dog longs for its owner.

All I want is for them to someday walk through my front door and *love me back.*

WE GET to the Benihana and it is packed.

It is clear that we are not the first dinner seating, nor are we the last of the lunch crowd. It is just wall-to-wall people.

Sharing tables with strangers and eating without masks on.

I'd put on a dress and make-up for the occasion, trying to lean into things, but as we're standing waiting for our table, my brother gave me some shit about masks, and I told him I'd take it off later. My dad's got a mask on, perhaps in solidarity, but it's underneath his nose, and I can feel the walls closing in.

And I don't want to ruin things, truly, because it's going to be an expensive meal, and I know my parents just wanted to take us all out someplace nice, but I'm feeling fragile—and I freaking told everyone, repeatedly, that it'd be my first time out at a restaurant in fifteen months—and then when they take us to our seats, I'm at the edge, near this couple and their little kid.

Have they been vaccinated? I sure as shit know that their two-year-old hasn't. What the fuck are they doing with their toddler out in public? And they're of an ethnicity that has higher death rates! My mind starts to spiral.

Then my brother lays in about unemployment, and Newsom's potential recall, and my parents agree—and he says, "And ten states are lifting their mask mandates shortly."

I try to have an opinion on this. I say that Newsom's been doing a good job and that California currently has the lowest positivity rating, which at the time it did.

My brother looks me in the eyes and says, "No they don't."

And that's what breaks me, and what I elided on Twitter for ease of explanation.

That I told him something that was true, and he went and shut me down.

I had sudden sinking realization of what the entire night was going to turn into. I snapped at him unprettily, I know, that he needed to shut up about covid right now or I would take a fucking Uber, and then I went into the bathroom and had my panic attack.

I didn't have anyone to back me up.

I was totally alone in this loud restaurant full of maskless people.

No one else there had any idea what I had been through or what last year was like, and no one cared, besides.

THAT'S UNFAIR, I know, because I've had those moments a lot in my life—where you experience something so grief-tacular that you can't shift back into the normal world, where you hate the normal world for being that way, angry that everyone else gets to go right on without you.

So I get that it's not everybody's job to recognize my trauma at all times. I'm not the center of the universe. I know.

BUT JUST DON'T FUCKING *lie* to me.

That's all I ask.

No more fucking lies.

I COME BACK, in tears, and I ask my brother if he'll go outside with me—all I want is the chance to explain to him how I feel, and what I've seen.

All I want is the chance to feel like his sister again.

But he says no, probably because he's freaked out by my crying. And then I say, "All I did last year was watch people die," with tears streaming down my cheeks, and he says something about how he just wanted to have a nice dinner.

Me too.

Me too.

Me too.

THE SHEER PHYSICALITY of loss is one thing. I can bathe another dead body if I have to. But looking someone in the eye who basically told me I was lying or shut me down as I tried to tell them my truth....

I sat back down on the bench by the unvaccinated child and put a straw into my soda with shaking hands.

5/1/21

I'm putting this out into the universe before I medicate myself to sleep: if any journalistic organization would like me to write a 3-5k essay on being a covid RN with PTSD trying to reintegrate with society, hit me up. I'm an amazing writer and I've given it a lot of thought. TY.

5/2/21

Hiding in the spare room at my parent's, "napping," i.e., trying not to cry.

Not sure how I'm going to manage the rest of this trip. T-minus 24 hrs.

I feel bad for them; they want the bright daughter they can be proud of, and instead they've just got me.

It's all fun and games to be proud of your nurse daughter, till she might tell you things you don't want to hear.

(Or she doesn't. Because there's no point. But at the same

time it makes her miserable to be unseen and unheard and un-understood.)

Not one person here has asked me about last year.

Not one.

And I guess maybe that's on me, too, I haven't exactly "gone there," with the exception of snapping at my mask-mocking brother yesterday.

Not a, "Hey, I bet that sucked," or. "Was it rough?"

Instead, I feel compelled to make myself smaller because the expansive version of me would swamp them all in a wave of sorrow.

I want to fit into the old person they were expecting, although let's be honest, she hasn't been around much since 2016.

I wish I could get my old family experience back.

When I felt safe, or at the least, freaking heard. When I thought these people cared for more than just my successes, but might be there for the bad parts, too.

But now I don't feel safe showing them the bad parts. I don't want to trust them with my vulnerability. I can't take the emotional blows of being gaslit right now, I really can't—and I'd have to pay $700 to Southwest to get me home tonight.

So I'll just keep "napping" and taking Ativan and gritting my teeth. I love them so much, and it kills me that they don't see what they're doing to me.

5/2/21

For people playing the home game, I am 2mg of Ativan in and am in bed now.

My brother came over and mostly hung with my folks.

Gave me a hug at the end. Said, "Thanks for keeping people alive," really fast, really quickly in my ear, so I guess he knows he was a dick yesterday?

Then he left and not even a large dose of benzos could keep my tongue still, so I told my parents everything, exactly like I promised my husband and other people I would not, and I guess crying was good. They're glad I'm getting help. They don't understand their culpability in why I need help.

I tried to explain just how much an "I'm sorry" would mean to me, but it just wasn't forthcoming.

Not really.

Not without a "but" after it, y'know.

So I continue to be their damaged daughter, who they love but take no ownership of their actions that led me to this point.

I remember, after Trump winning, crying on the phone with my mother, trying to explain how much she'd boned me, a nurse, and my husband, a Jewish man who fights for broadband equity/net neutrality. How she put both our lives and livelihoods in danger.

She didn't get it then, and she doesn't get it now.

It's not a calloused not getting it... it's just an inability to 360-view things, due to soaking in Republicanism for so long.

For instance, my folks no longer watch NBA games, after having been huge fans for decades.

I said, yeah, because of racism.... Whereas she's just "disgusted by all the politics" in sports now.

She just can't bridge that gap.

Completely unable to see it. But if Greg Popovich can't stop my folks from being racist after they've worshipped at the church of the Spurs forever.... [CA: Greg Popovich is the coach of the Spurs and was the first coach to comment positively on the BLM movement, if I recall correctly.]

So I've done all I could do. At least I was honest with them. And I can go back to protecting myself tomorrow.

I was told they feel like they have to walk on eggshells

around me, because I call them out on racist/classist stuff—
they don't get that I also feel like that with them.

I'll fly away, and they'll go back to intensely praying for
me, their brain-case daughter, at their church that's
apparently OK with letting half-a-million people die of covid,
and never once will an iota of hypocrisy get through to them.

They're so aggrieved. Because of me making them feel
awkward in the past. And "this world isn't our world" and
"this world is going to hell" Jesus-stuff.

I'm sorry, I didn't see Jesus lift a single finger last year in
the ICU. Not a damn one.

I was looking for Him, really hard. He had several
chances to pull off a miracle for me.

The bar in 2020 was really fucking low.

Anyhow.

I'm about to Ambien out. I don't know how to process this
ill-fitting love. It's like being in a dressing room with an outfit
you last wore when you were twelve. I wish I could get back
into it and have those feels again.

But I've been too sharp for too long. I've hurt them and
they've hurt me, and it just is what it is now, whatever this
may be.

I had to listen to my brother talk about unemployment
being "too high" last night at dinner, which I called him out
on, because JFC, he has an effing Porsche. He wants for
nothing, he thinks he deserves it, and that Jesus is on his side...
and I know my parents are.

It's just... everything's unfair. I know that's true and
always has been, on a base level, I've seen it all, good people
dying horribly, and vice versa. I don't wish him nor my
parents ill.

But goddamn, do I wish I could give them all just one
drop of empathy.

~╷┴╷┴╷┴╷~

AND THIS IS when the hot takes about "whether people are cling-ingly fearfully to masks?" begin.

To every journalist who thought that it was appropriate to write an article, do an interview, or post an Op Ed that even began to coun-tenance that idea—fuck you.

Heartily. Sideways. In the neck.

Did you need to carry water for the half of America that is still okay with everyone else dying? Was it important that when they handed you their shotgun, you loaded it up with ammo?

Fuck. You.

I'M sure it felt real exciting at the time, sitting there in front of your computer, your kids screeching somewhere behind you, you having been home, safe, since the beginning of the pandemic, no skin in the game.

You were all, "Here's my chance. I'm gonna zing 'em! Devil's advocate, ahoy!"

The devil needs no more advocates, asshole.

What the fuck.

"Are masks maladaptive?" you asked, when over three fourths of the country still wasn't vaccinated.

Only if I'm shoving one down your throat so you don't say idiotic things.

5/6/21

Mental health update: my psychiatrist doubled my meds on Tues. Picked 'em up today, will be trying them out tomorrow.

My out-of-pocket therapist couldn't see me today. She

had a family emergency, and I'm not sure when she'll be back. My current health insurance has yet to find me one.

5/11/21

I'm overly invested in my dove niece/nephew here. They should hatch any day now....

5/12/21

For the record, my health insurance has yet to assign me a therapist.

I told them that I now have a month off, my schedule's free, and still nothing. I talk to my old out-of-pocket therapist tomorrow. What's everyone else supposed to do?

When the mental health reckoning for healthcare workers lands, there's not going to be anyone.

5/13/21

I wrote 100,000 words in two months. Hypergraphia's a kiss and a curse. I wish I hadn't been so monofocused on writing for a bit. It probably wasn't good for my mental health.

But when my mental health was bad, having someplace I could go that made me happy made all the difference.

5/13/21

My therapist: On a scale from 1-10, where ten is suicidal, how depressed are you?

Me: Dr. S, perhaps a better question would be, have I ever been happy?

5/13/21

DOVELINGS!!! The momma flew off and I caught a quick snap!!!

We're going to our first party with all our friends who've been vaccinated tomorrow, and my husband is all, "Remember, honey, some people have been drinking all pandemic. If you try to stay caught up, your liver might die."

Based on comparing year over year excess mortality numbers, scientists now believe that the American death total is over 900,000 people. (5/13/21)

5/15/21

Had a real, non-traumatic lunch out with my BFF in person, who got me to level with her, regarding all my recent life and trauma, and halfway through I turned on my phone's voice recorder....

Because I'm going to finish the book I'm working on in three-four days—and then I'm going write my covid-nursing book. [CA: this book! Right here!]

My therapist says it's a good idea. I'm a fast writer, and I already have skads of material from Two Nurses Talking. Even if I have to self-pub it, that's fine. I probably already have 30k of material, honestly.

I really am going to do this. All my closest friends at this party tonight agree.

Right now I'm a little tipsy, drunk on true friendship, vodka cranberries, and the power of maybe, just maybe getting to release.

I know how to debride a wound and heal it whole again.

THIS PARTY WAS the first time I'd gotten to see most of my oldest best friends in person in fifteen months.

I know they saw each other some from appropriate distances during that time—but because of where I was working, and who I was working with, it didn't feel right for me to hang out and put anyone else in danger.

But that day, that glorious day, I got to walk into my friend's house—it felt like coming home, because it was.

I got to give each of them the world's best longest hug, and I only got tearful once, starting to sob, "You all lived. You all lived!" but then I got even more hugs, and everything was all right.

My husband and I got to hang out on their back porch, held in their love as we held them back, trading stories and hopes again, and I finally, for the slightest bit, began to feel like I was going back to normal.

The sweetest and best part about that party though, was that all along, all of my friends had listened to me. Really, they were so smart and with it that they would've been fine without me. But just knowing that they were each being as safe as they possibly could all along, so that they were going to make it through—I never had to worry about them putting themselves in danger. I never had to hope that they'd make it out all right.

I got to drink—something I didn't let myself do the entire pandemic, because alcohol's a depressant and clearly I needed no help—I got to spend the night in someone else's bed, and wake up to someone else cooking bacon.

It was amazing.

THE WEEK after that I really Concentrated on Getting Better, using the tools I had at my disposal and my prior experiences with myself. I saw other people in person every single day, I exercised every day, I spent time in my garden every day... and it didn't help.

I wasn't suicidal anymore, yeah, but I also wasn't whole, and the thought of having to go into work again made me want to cry and throw up. I figured I had PTSD, just based on my vague knowledge of it from books and movies, but I hadn't done any of those tests online because I didn't really want to know.

I have a hard time admitting that I'm broken. (Shush, I am. It's true.) And I don't need to be "beautifully" broken or any other empowering weirdness that tries to make it sound like this is a good thing to have happened.

I just don't want to be like this. Really.

And I find it frustrating, too, that mental health is an experience on a continuum, you know?

Like, if someone came into the hospital with sepsis, *boom*, I'd know what to do to do. Things might get sketchy, but if I performed These Certain Rituals, with my tools and medications, one of the outcomes would be that You'll Get Better.

Whereas with brain stuff... I don't really know.

I am different now.

I will always be different.

I want to get better, but there's no guarantees, and I find that terrifying. And even when my brain gets better, which I sincerely hope it will, I will still have scars.

So I was just kind of ignoring things, but my therapist made me take an official test, and I'll go through a sampling of questions from a generic version, so you know what it's like:

IN THE PAST MONTH, have you had:

    1. Nightmares?

Somehow, I manage to have nightmares on Ambien, which is quite a triumph of my brain's desire to fuck with me.

The worst of the most recent ones that stuck with me was this: I was in a dark room, taking care of a patient, and they were infested with ants. I was trying to convince them to get treatment, but they kept refusing, and I was getting increasingly distressed. They let me touch them, and so I touched part of their thigh and it crumbled off of them, revealing more ants beneath, tunneling through their flesh. I showed this to them and it didn't matter, they wouldn't let me help them. There was still nothing I could do.

2. Felt numb or detached.

Yes. Very, very yes.

I (used to) disassociate all the time. (It's better now, here in June.)

If you're lucky enough not to know what that's like, let me try to explain it—for me it's like when a grey fog permeates my entire being. It's kind of like being in "the well," but it doesn't always mean I don't want to live.

I just feel disconnected from things. Like I could move right through them, and them through me. Everything blends together, and there's no joy to be had. Or really any anger.

I'm just there. Being. Breathing. But not really "alive."

3. Intrusive images or memories of events?

I was watching a show last week, online, with a friend, and a character on that show died at a hospital, and they found out because the doctor came out to tell them they'd "done all they could," and you have no idea how triggering that was for me.

I was crying so hard on my couch that my husband, who'd been at work up in his office with the door closed, came down to check on me.

Just the feeling of utter helplessness that that evoked, remembering what it was like to talk to so many families, all wanting the same impossible thing that I couldn't give them—good news—it was just like being there again. It was heart wrenching.

4. Angry, or other emotional outbursts.

Well, fucking clearly.

5/18/21

Before I went to sleep, momma dove and baby dove were nesting.

This morning, they're both gone and now poppa dove is flying around my deck looking for them, calling.

I'm going back to plants where things don't die.

My husband says I shouldn't look for external validation in keeping things alive, as far as doves are concerned at least, but it's stupidly hitting me pretty hard.

I'm crying now.

I still have two weeks off before work again.

What if I don't get better?

AND SO I started this book.

Because writing/collating a book about a year's worth of trauma is one hundred percent a me-thing to do.

One of my friends gave me that book, *The Body Keeps the Score*. I'll be honest, I haven't read it yet, but I already know it's premise is true.

The grey rape incident with my ex happened on New Year's Eve, and let me tell you, while I'm sure there's never a good time for bad things to happen, it really fucking sucks when they happen on national holidays.

I used to go pretty crazy every NYE and I didn't put it together until I started dating my now husband, who was all, "Uh, yeah, is this your permanent setting?" Which made me reflect, for the first time, on why I was doing what I was doing, and I pinned it back to that moment and realized that subconsciously it was huge and occupied far more territory inside my psyche than I was giving it credit for.

After that, I made it a point to go out with friends and do strongly good, happy, fun things on NYE, to reclaim it in a way, and I like to think that now I fully have.

I'm relating this story to you all so you might consider now what it might be like to have lived through 365-plus days of bad things happening. Witnessing the deaths, feeling the despair.

What do you do when your trauma isn't something that can be self-contained to a discrete period in time? When, for an entire year, the majority of your days were bad?

How do you begin to process that, and how can you hope to heal?

Especially when the societal reaction to all I and other nurses have gone through seems to have been... silence?

You have to acknowledge that there's a problem, for there to be a solution. And the way we're being treated now wraps me into Nurses Week.

Let me tell you a meme that was making the rounds Nurses Week 2021: it's a photo of a little girl at a desk, holding her head and crying as she attempts to write.

The caption?

"When the shitty pen you got for Nurses Week breaks while you're writing your suicide note."

This is what passes for humor on nurse boards.

And yes, we all are morbid fucks. We have to be, to survive—but surely you can read between the lines.

One of my close nursing friends, her management told them, "You all need to stop joking about killing yourselves!" without the slightest hint of self-awareness, as the staffing ratios they approved at her ED slowly ground her and others like her into dust.

NURSES ARE AT SIGNIFICANTLY HIGHER risk of suicide than the general populace.

Among a general female population, there's 8.6 suicides per 100,000.

Among female nurses?

17.1.

OUR STATS WERE HIGH, even pre-pandemic—mostly because the general population doesn't realize what the for-profit healthcare system has been increasingly asking of us for decades now.

You see, we really are trying to take care of you.

But corporations? The people that run healthcare? The people that don't touch you or talk to you on the phone?

By and large?

They don't give a shit.

They don't care if we get breaks or have opportunities to take vacations. They don't care if we get to keep our retirements or pensions. They don't care if we break ourselves physically, emotionally, mentally, trying to care for you.

You know how we can tell? Because other thrilling Nurses Week gifts across the country included (in several locations!) nurses getting rocks, along with little letters saying, "Nurses Rock!"—I shit you not.

So upper management just trusts in us to continue to do the right thing—i.e., not letting people die, trying to provide good care with respect and dignity—under increasingly stressful conditions, despite the lingering psychic damage of last year, because that's what we've always done—and if we stop doing it, they think they can hire someone else to do it.

And this current contradiction between a management that doesn't care about their staff on site but who yet seem capable of endlessly overpaying for travelers to fill in gaps makes about as much sense as shooting your own dick off. (Again, no hate on travelers; I definitely hate the game, not the players.)

It only works if view our occupation sheerly though a capitalist lens, as it's so obvious most healthcare management does, because since 2016, the average hospital turned over 83% of their RN workforce, due to a combination of churn and burn at the lower end of the experience scale, and older RNs retiring out. Those of us sandwiched in the middle, trying to hold down the fort, are dying.

Sometimes literally.

HERE'S THE THING, too—once people we like, trust, and enjoy leave the floor—there's absolutely no reason for us to stay behind without them.

It only takes a few strong nurses deciding to retire or abandon ship for an entire floor's safety-net of knowledge and morale to unravel like a cheap sweater. There are people whose presences anchor a floor, and once they leave, all that experience and goodwill is walking out with them.

Let met set this off with a paragraph break:

YOUR FLOOR IS ONLY AS GOOD AS THE CUMULATIVE KNOWLEDGE OF ALL YOUR NURSES ON IT AT ANY TIME.

. . .

I CANNOT EMPHASIZE enough for laypeople how important experience-in-nursing is to actual-nursing. And while, yes, everyone needs to start somewhere, if your nurses don't know what they don't know—which is a very common thing, for your first few years of nursing—you're toast.

To be a good nurse, you need to be humble enough to ask for help —but you also need to be smart enough to know when you *need* to ask for help.

We all made fun of Donald Rumsfeld's "unknown unknowns" back in the day, but that's actually (I cannot believe I'm going to say this about a member of the GOP) a good way to look at it.

If you do not know what you don't know—if the breadth of experiences you've gained on your floor hasn't fully encompassed yet what you *need* to know—there's a very good chance that your patients could slip through those cracks, through no fault of yours!

But in addition to knowing what you don't know—you need to be in an environment where asking for help is actually going to produce answers.

If a hospital can't retain good people, it almost by definition cannot hire good people. Why would a good nurse—especially in these times—subject themselves to poor pay or poor management at a facility where they won't feel safe and supported in their patient care? What nurse of experience and good conscience wants to roll in and be the anchor on a new-grad/new-hire floor?

Sure, there are competent people who just keep their heads down and do their jobs... but at this stage in the hospital staffing game, if you're mobile, those type of people are likely going elsewhere as travelers to cash out, because they don't need those personal attachments to friends or a facility to feel fulfilled.

And if you're working at a facility where staff is leaving like rats abandoning a sinking ship, chances are you're going to leave, too.

We do not roll into work to make management happy.

We did not risk our lives for all of 2020 to save people, at least on the ICU, once we started realizing, hey, we probably couldn't.

We kept coming to work because we trusted in, believed in, and wanted to help our coworkers.

We were saving each other in 2020 because we had to.

BENEFITS ARE GREAT, and pay's nice too—but at the end of the day, everyone wants to be happy to go into work, and feel happy leaving it. Everyone wants to have a sense of accomplishment, and more than that, as nurses we need it.

This may sound childish to you, because you think, of course not everyone likes their job—but consider that when we don't like our jobs, people fucking die! I guarantee you no nurse in the US wants to go home and wonder if they did something that might've led to a patient's demise. No one wants to question the skills or safety of the people they work with, or question management's intent in staffing them poorly every. Single. Day.

We need the camaraderie of our coworkers who're in the trenches with us to see us through.

And if our beloved coworkers leave—and if they leave with cause, like so many are right now, seeing as we all feel equally disposable— there is no reason for us not to leave with them.

MY OLD MANAGER getting fired felt like a punch in the gut—right before the covid holidays, too. I don't want to get too specific, lest I get outed, but it sure did feel like (barring any other communication from managers On High) he was getting punished for protecting us and our staffing ratios during the first wave, and also for giving us overtime.

I trusted him. I'd banked points with him, and he with me. If he texted me personally, I knew it was a choice between me coming in or him literally being on the floor and helping us, because that's the kind of manager he was.

I respected him, because I knew that he was in the trenches with me.

Every single position he opened up prior to getting fired at my facility is STILL CURRENTLY OPEN. (All that teaching you saw me do above was on-boarding travelers, not actual 'going to really stay here now' hires.)

And it's not because we're not paying well, because hello, it's California money (even though California is still a pricey place to live.)

They literally cannot get qualified staff to apply.

And now, without him there, to for me to keep coming in when we're always short and not getting breaks and don't have competent management—it's June! We still don't have a real replacement manager!—I wouldn't be "banking points" with anyone.

I'd essentially be enabling my own abuse.

Because until I and other nurses stop picking up extra shifts, at my hospital and so many others, upper management will never learn —even though in the act of not taking those shifts, I hurt my coworkers, who deserve to pee and eat, and also myself, in that my scheduled shifts will be equally low on help.

It fucking sucks that we're being expected to pick up the slack for poor management, to the detriment of ourselves and our coworkers— and more than that—***it's not right.***

So—what can be done?

Well, let me start small and work my way up.

For people that work in the hospital:

If you're a manager reading this, give your nurses more autonomy and more ability to be in charge of their own schedules, create more part-time positions that allow flexibility for childcare, and hire more RNs. Give appreciation both verbally and in written formats. Participate in hospital-wide recognition activities as well as the Daisy award. If you are short staffed on the floor, get out there and help. Give a break or two or help with a turn. Deflect that angry family member's attention. Give hazard pay and make sure adequate PPE is ALWAYS AVAILABLE. Give nurses parking passes for your facility—no nurse should ever have to pay to park, what the fuck nonsense is that? Be present, as much as you can—and if you feel all of this is too much of a drain on you, on top of your already busy duties, then consider that you, too, are being taken advantage of and maybe you too should agitate for change at higher levels (or leave). Perhaps you need an assistant manager. But don't you dare roll your shit downhill onto floor nurses—they've already got enough going on. If you can't be a proactive, positive management force in their lives, then why are you there? If you aren't trying to protect your employees' physical and mental livelihoods, then what are you doing?

And above all else: NEVER FORGET WHAT IT FEELS LIKE TO WORK ON THE FLOOR.

Let me repeat: NEVER, EVER, FORGET WHAT IT FEELS LIKE TO WORK ON THE FLOOR.

Just because you get to roll up to the hospital in nicer clothing and you don't have to lay your hands on a bath wipe doesn't mean that you're better than any of us. It just means that you chose a different path.

You need to respect us, so that we can in turn respect you, and we can *all* do what is best for our patients.

And if, somehow, you're in management over nurses and you've never had to physically *be* a nurse? For shame, really—and my temptation is to ask, "who the fuck do you think you are?"—but that still doesn't give you an excuse to treat us like commodities.

We are people, dammit.

And we're not nearly as replaceable as you think we are.

If you want to create a low-turnover culture where you get to keep experienced nurses on hand, which has been statistically shown to have better outcomes for patients—which is, ostensibly, why we're all here—we need to feel valued and we need to be protected.

Which brings me to unions.

Let your nurses unionize.

No, not all nursing unions are perfect, but at the end of the day, most nurses are going to feel their interests are far more safeguarded when they've got a union at their back. That isn't to say that management can't be a force for good; they can... it's just so often they choose not to be.

I've heard horror stories online about how, when other nurses were in nursing school, they actually had someone come in and run a "nurses' unions are bad!" day.

But let me tell you what unions have accomplished out in California—we're the only state that has a staffing ratio law.

Why?

Because our unions worked, and worked hard, to get it and to keep it.

Apparently only 20% of nurses feel staffing is safe at their hospital, and most of them are in California, I'm assuming.

If I have not convinced you that nurses work hard already, let me now try a different tack.

Surely you have met a toddler or two in your time—so imagine trying to keep an eye on two toddlers, in two separate rooms, trying to keep them out of trouble, without tying them to the bed or sedating them to sleep. This should sound fairly hard to you, if you have met toddlers.

Now... try to imagine keeping five-to-eight toddlers safe all at once, in separate rooms, or out in the open, in hallways, like some emergency departments have to.

This should strike you as nigh impossible.

If you're all, "but patients aren't toddlers!" clearly you have never met someone with Alzheimer's, who spends the whole shift shouting for their dead husband and trying to fall out of bed, someone detoxing who is in the process of gnawing their way through their restraints, or someone we're attempting to wean off of sedation to extubate safely, who has no idea what-the-fuck has happened to them or why they're in the hospital or how they got there, who is thrashing around like they're an extra in the Exorcist—and that's before we get to the patients who are inpatient at the hospital because of cardiac events or organ failure.

No, not all floors are inundated with critical patients simultaneously, but... *come on....*

It doesn't take a genius to see that better staffing ratios equals better outcomes, because OF COURSE IT DOES.

Will that mean that you need to hire more nurses? Possibly! And that's OK!

Let's not go into this with a scarcity mentality, because when we look at hospital administration's salaries... they've got room to share.

Did the decisions the CEO of my hospital system made mean that they should make—and I did the math—42 times what I do?

Did they save 42 times as many people as me?

Did they watch 42 times as many people die?

I feel pretty confident that if we turned my hospital system's C-suite types over and shook out their pockets, you could hire an extra nurse or two for my floor and all the others with the change.

[CA: I'm writing this from California, where I do get paid pretty fairly/well—but across the nation, in hospitals without unions, there are nurses working far harder than I am, with far worse staffing ratios, for half the pay. If you don't want all of your nurses to come out to California as travelers, the rest of the US is going to need to step up in a big way.]

Outside of the hospital:

If you're reading this and you're not a healthcare person, we need you to wake the fuck up. (You might already be awake, but there hasn't been much cursing in this section, thus far.)

Stop voting for assholes who don't care if you live or die.

If anyone ever tries to politicize public health again, from here on out, know that that person needs to be deplatformed instantaneously. Take away their microphones, take away their funding, and change the channel.

There is no time nor place for playing devil's advocate when lives are on the line.

And? There is no level of preventable death that is statistically "okay."

It's not okay for people to die who didn't have to, and it's not okay for you to expect someone else to have to watch those deaths, either.

Recognize that healthcare is a right and that everyone should have access to it.

Get your vaccines, as soon as you can, and if this one needs boosters, those too.

If you belong to an organized religion that says that it's okay that people die, reconsider your church affiliation immediately. And I'm sorry if realizing that "it's not okay if people die" leads you to other such mind-blowing conclusions as we ought to feed the hungry and house the homeless. Yes, those things are also true.

And if taxes on rich people or corporate taxes have to increase to make that happen? All the fucking better.

I'll never forget a conversation my mom had with my husband, where she was worried about the death tax because Fox News had told her it was an important thing and she didn't want all her money to go to the government... whereupon my husband asked her, "Do you have assets worth more than five million dollars?" To which the answer was, of course, "No."

She was worried about something that would never affect her, all because Fox News wanted her to vote to protect rich people.

Look, when's the last time a rich person ever did a thing for you? Honestly. Meaningful billionaire philanthropy is a myth. I think the Gates Foundation making sure that covid vaccines were patented rather than open source should be the pin that pops that balloon once and for all. They did reverse their course, but not until MAY OF 2021. *Jesus.*

And last, but not least: turn off Fox news.

Turn off Fox news.

Turn off Fox news.

WHETHER YOU LIKE it or not, we live in a society. It is comprised of all of us individuals, and we are only as collectively healthy as the least of us, really—but you cannot keep banking on breaking nurses to support you under these conditions.

We've been through enough. We're over it.

We shouldn't have to be *this fucking strong.*

I KNOW to some degree this entire book I've been preaching, or shouting, at the choir—mostly so I can get all these thoughts out of my head and onto the page—but if I do publish this and you do wind up reading it—the second you start seeing hit pieces come out in six months about the "Upcoming Nursing Shortage!" or "Hospitals Don't Have Enough Staff!" I want you to think about everything I've written here.

I can already tell from looking at the past and how we were treated during covid—and how we're seeing service workers being treated now—that people are going to write snarky shit like, "What do they need more money for? They should be grateful they have a job!"

And we'll point to ourselves, to our experiences, to all of last year, and some dumbfuck is going to say, "But you're a nurse! You should be used to seeing people die!"

And to that singular future person, I say this, "No. No one should *ever* have to get used to seeing people die. And if your nurse *is* used to seeing people die—you want a different nurse."

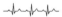

MY HEALTH INSURANCE'S "employee assistance program" finally "found" me an in-network therapist on 5/21. I got ahold of her and she wanted to know what was going on. I told her I knew I had PTSD, that I was having problems regulating my emotions, and I started crying.

And she... started to pull back.

I have a sixth sense for people pulling away. I definitely have abandonment issues, which leads to me not putting myself out there a lot of the time, except for on paper. And, uh, maybe that's why I put myself out there on paper so much, come to think on it. I'm a real person, and I'll do real-people things, but I don't like to let myself get hurt by someone leaving me, so I just don't often truly connect unless I'm really feeling it.

But I felt helpless in that moment.

All I want to do in life is to get better, right? I don't want to live with this current version of me, the one that sees something sad on TV or has something sad happen in real life, who breaks down sobbing, uncontrollably—this pathetic meatshell I'm trapped inside of now, who currently can't hack it.

So I start sobbing that I'm not that crazy, which, as you can imagine, was a super-effective maneuver, and she artfully says she only has an opening every other week, and that I sound like an "I need therapy every week" kind of girl.

It was like getting cruised on a coffee shop first date by the person you knew you were supposed to be meeting, and seeing them walk off without even sitting down.

After she got off the phone with me, having promised that she'd call my health insurance back to explain that she couldn't take me on —that it was "her" not "me," despite how much "me" it felt as I sat there, sobbing. I just felt lost.

I am super lucky that I do have my old therapist—and I've given up on finding a new one for free. I'm just paying out of pocket now, ride or die—but, like, how do other people do this, who aren't me? Who don't have a backup in their pocket?

It was so funny, too, prior to that, when I'd called in initially and then asked, every other day, if they'd found anyone to assign to me yet —I didn't know I was going to get time off, and so they kept asking what time I could meet, and I couldn't say. My work schedule looks like someone's sneezed on a calendar, right? I don't always have off every other Tuesday, because inpatient nursing doesn't often work like that. And then they'd ask me, "Well, can you just get an hour off? Or call in on your lunch break?"

And what I wanted to say to that was, "I'm an ICU nurse. You think I get a whole hour off? And do you think I know when the hell —and if!—my lunch break will be?"

What I'm saying is that healthcare workers are so screwed.

(And also that, if you've seen a therapist before, now's the time to reach out, before they get super booked.)

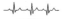

5/26/21—private slack with friends

I'm having a very "Oh nooooooooo" type morning here regarding this project.

I keep getting scared it'll make my family mad.

Which is partially why I committed and got the preorder up now and hyped it so that I Can't Back Out Now.

But some part of me just wishes we could all get along.

Some tiny childish part.

I just want them to see things my way, and they literally never will. And I feel bad for that part of me because she's so scared all the time, and I don't think I can ever really set her free.

I just appreciate having a place to talk about it and be sad and scared in turns, J. I'm really going to take y'all up on this whole "safe space channel" thing, heh.

I went out to coffee yesterday with a friend, and she was telling me how close she and her dad are, and I wanted to burst into tears because I don't think I'll ever have that again, but we really did used to be!

In many ways, my life is so, so good. I've got great friends and found family.

I just miss what I once had.

If I'd never have had it, this wouldn't hurt so bad, you know?

And so sometimes I just get swept with this great and overwhelming sadness, one there's no fix for, other than just not thinking about it, I guess, and that makes me sad, too. I once felt like I could rely on my brother for anything, and my parents always had my back, and now I just know that's not the case.

No matter how many friends love you, it's just not the same.

They fit into different slots inside your soul.

5/26/21—password protected journal

Still cranking away on my nurse book. I've got a lot of pre-orders now (thanks, y'all! <3) so that's good, and my therapist actually turned in my leave paperwork for through 8/1, which means I could have all summer off.

I find that astounding.

Good-capitalist-drone-Cassie freaked out about that yesterday. I mean, that's more downtime than I've ever-ever had, since summer break between nursing school years.

At the same time... I really do need it. Like I was telling her, I feel like all the boxes I've been shoving shit into are burping open, and I don't know how to fix that, you know? I feel like my choices are either drill the lids back down, or write this book—a book which, by its very nature, is going to make certain people unhappy, which makes me anxious—and open all the boxes and set everything inside them free.

It definitely feels like a "the only way out is through" thing.

5/26/21—author newsletter

Hello from Cassie, RN!

Hi everybody! I know I've been quiet for a long stretch here... and I never know how to start things like this, so here goes: personal information up top, and book news below.

First off—I've been diagnosed with PTSD related to working at the hospital last year, and I'm home from work right now.

I'm not entirely sure when I'll be going back to work—probably much, much later in the summer, when I've had the chance to build up some resilience, which for me would mean going for 72 hrs. without crying.

I mean—I do want to go back. Being a nurse is who I am, every bit as much as being a writer.

But I can't go back if I can't get my shit under control. I mean, I kind of want to cry just writing this.

I spent so long being strong while being scared last year that I feel like I've run out of strength now, for myself. I don't have anything left to give—even though I don't have to be scared now, not anymore. But I can't turn that part off so easily, either. It's like it's baked in there too.

Needless to say, I'm in therapy, and we're changing my psych meds some, under medical supervision.

Anyhow... I've never met a trauma I haven't tried to write

through, you know? So while I'm here, sitting on my couch and mostly not crying, I've started a new book that I put up for pre-order. It's called *Year of the Nurse*.

Nurses will recognize that phrase with irony, because the World Health Organization designated 2020 as the Year of the Nurse, so we got to think, "Yeah, fucking right," a lot, last year (or maybe just if you were me).

I kept a lot of journals last year, and you all know I sent you newsletters explaining things, and I tweeted a bunch—this book's going to be a collated version of everything that happened to me, chronologically, with some additional thoughts from me, now.

It's also going to be very, very angry, which is why I haven't shared the link yet. I wanted to warn you first. I'm still mad that last year happened the way it did, when it didn't have to. I'm mad that serving a mad king "broke" me.

But mostly I'm mad that so many people died who didn't have to.

So—it's not going be an uplifting book, although there will be moments of levity in it, and gear shifts from white-hot anger to informative scientific explanations about how the hospital works and what it's like to be an ICU nurse.

But if you're mad about last year too, and you want to feel some catharsis in not being alone in that—or if you want to know what being a nurse last year really felt like, up close and personal, this book may be the book for you, or for a nurse friend, or other interested parties.

I set its pre-order for October because I wanted to give myself some room, but I'm very sure I'll have it done by August.

So that's what's up and new with me. I'm just trying to get by. It's hard for me to acknowledge that there's anything wrong with me because I don't want there to be, you know? Who wants to have a broken brain? And in some ways, I still function well—I can drive, I can go to the grocery store, and words are still my refuge. I just don't know if I can handle seeing anyone die again.

I wish I could go out on some snappy finger-gun type thing

because, Christ, I am literally the world's worst Marketer of Things—but also, my ability to lie, or indeed give a shit about lying, is at a personal all-time low. So I suspect these are the weirdest author newsletters you receive, heh. Sorry.

More soon, when another book comes out,

<3

Cassie

[CA: in response to this, a reader sent me a photo of her husband and daughter, who she said I helped to keep safe last year, and I cried for a million years. Good tears, though, at least, at last.]

JUNE 2021

On June 3rd, one of my coworker-friends reached out to me to make sure I hadn't quit. Several coworkers have reached out with equal concern during this time off, but I've been very vague about why I'm gone and am just claiming family stuff, because I don't want to be seen as "crazy." It's silly, because they all are truly awesome. I just don't want to talk about things really, until I get back —whereupon I'm sure I will, because I'm compulsively honest.

It turns out my friend had also had time "off" and after beating around the bush a bit, we both confessed that we'd been taking mental health breaks.

She's in gray, on the left, I'm in blue on the right:

It took me a while to finally let myself fall apart, to be. I was so broken I didn't know where to start to fix myself

I spent like three weeks crying at dumb shit, lolsob

and I don't know if I'm getting fixed or just putting lids back on all the tupperwares full of shit in my head

heh

how did you get better?

You're sorting through it. Getting rid of the containers without life and such

i keep thinking i'm better then finding out i'm not

Lids

It's a process. I went to the beach a lot

nodnod

Therapy

Trying to figure out how the pre-covid and post covid life are going to blend together here on out.

That one I'm struggling with now

how so?

We won't ever go back to our pre covid lives.

yeah

the scabs are pulled off, and the rocks yanked up

And this post covid life scarred us. Especially health care. We've learned how horrible people can truly be.

yeah

SO MUCH YEAH

i get so ANGRY still

and I don't know what to do with that

So trying to find this happy medium to move forward

> i want to honor it, right, because, it's earnest

> but at the same time i can't walk around like a bomb all the time

Lots of soul searching and making peace. It won't ever go away but it will lessen

IS SHE RIGHT?
I don't know.
I do hope so, though.

JULY 2021

Today is July 5th and I think this book is through.

I SENT it out for copyedits last week and I just approved the last of them today (so any grammar errors from here on out are mine). I have professional people making a cover for me, and I'm even trying to figure out an audiobook angle, if I can manage to narrate it all myself without crying.

I've been continuing therapy. We've been doing EMDR-style-stuff, like what they do with combat vets, and that has been quite helpful.

Perhaps more helpful than that though has been sheer time: time away from the hospital to gain distance, and time to put this book together here.

I really think I might be able to manage going back to work at the end of this month, and I attribute that to all the processing I got to do inside these pages.

If I hadn't worked so hard on this book, letting it obsess me for a month and a half, going through twice as much material as I wound up actually including—and holding those individual memories up to the light, actually letting myself feel them at long last, acknowledging the things that happened to me in the open, out loud—I don't think I would have ever found my way back.

Not to the bedside, and maybe even not to myself.

Which isn't to say that I'm fixed and shit, just that it's finally within the realm of possibility.

BEING AN AUTHOR IS, in its own way, just as strange a calling as being a nurse.

You have to believe in a book with all of your heart and give it all of your effort, without attaching any value to whether or not it will succeed.

And once a book is out there, it is on its own.

It might sink or swim, but reader reaction to it is entirely out of your control.

I won't even know if you actually made it to this page.

But I hope you have, now that I'm not pretending you don't exist anymore, future reader. And I so wonder what is in store for the both of us.

Right now as I'm writing this, the Delta variant is ripping its way through the world. It is the dominant strain in California currently. The Midwest is getting pummeled, and hospitals there are putting out SOS calls for respiratory therapists.

People are still dying of covid who didn't have to *every day.*

Each covid death, from here on out now that we know better, and especially in the US because we have easy access to vaccines, is entirely preventable.

Are we going to splinter into two Americas, the vaccinated and the non? Those who understand the science and those who disregard it to their detriment? The irony is not lost on me that the same people who aren't getting vaccinated are the same people who vote Republican, and they'll go onto become the same people who won't have good access to future medical care for their covid-survivor symptoms *because* they voted Republican.

Can we get everyone on board with science before we accidentally create another, worse, disease?

I don't really know, though I wish I did, so badly, for us both.

BUT MY JOB here was just to tell you what last year was like for me– that's all I promised going in—and I like to think I accomplished that.

I won't lie, working on anything akin to a 'memoir' has felt ridiculously self-indulgent, which has sometimes made working on this project hard.

But any time I got scared about the enormity of that though, I thought of two things:

First, that Mike Pence—AKA the "Christian Cadaver," according to my biodad—got a seven-figure book deal.

I spent the past year pumping my brain and soul like a bellows, trying to keep everyone I knew alive, whereas he did... what? I mean, the man oversaw that HIV crisis in Indiana as governor and wrote pro-smoking op-eds in college. He wouldn't recognize a public health initiative if it bit him on the ass and handed him a business card. If he deserves a no-doubt ghostwritten book, then surely I deserve a real one.

And secondly, since someone's going to write a book about all this mess—it might as well be me.

I don't want anyone else telling—or co-opting—my story.

I know my experiences may not have been universal—even when I may have grandiosely made it seem like they were.

But they were *mine*. This is how I felt, straight up, this whole damn time. I didn't change any of my experiences or feelings.

This book is how it was for *me*.

. . .

IN THE END, the only thing I am absolutely sure of is that I never want to have to write another book like this again.

So don't make me, okay?

You already know what you need to do, having read this far, so I'm not going to repeat myself.

Just promise me that this past year of my life—*of all of our lives*—**especially the 600,000-plus who died**—wasn't totally for nothing.

Because if we can't learn lessons from the past, then we truly don't deserve a future.

All nurses, everywhere, only want to save lives.

Please stop fighting public health.

Stay safe,

<3

Cassie

(7/5/21)

CASSANDRA ALEXANDER IS a nurse of fourteen years, and a paranormal romance author. For more information about this book and others, you can visit her website at http://www.cassiealexander.com. She has a separate mailing list for people interested in Year of the Nurse: http://www.cassiealexander.com/yon-list

THE BIBLIOGRAPHY and citations for all of my news sources follows.

BIBLIOGRAPHY

I'm going to get to the Year of the Nurse's bibliography, but first – I really want you to look at and read these two articles. I promise they're both good and very worthwhile. Go check them out, and then you can come back to peruse my citations and additional commentary. (As you are reading the print edition, I'm sorry these links aren't 'live' for you.)

DEFOREST, ANNA. "THE WORLD'S GREATEST." The Paris Review, 16 Dec. 2020, https://www.theparisreview.org/blog/2020/12/16/the-heros/.

DR. DEFOREST WRITES *one million times* more eloquently than me, and she absolutely captured what it was like to be there. An utter must read.

    And—

· · ·

GRAY, Nathan. "Before the Pandemic, U.S. Healthcare Already Had a Crisis. . ." Medium, 27 Apr. 2020, https://nathan-gray10.medium.com/before-the-pandemic-u-s-healthcare-already-had-a-crisis-bdfd1751afa0.

DR. GRAY DREW a beautiful cartoon about how broken healthcare in America truly is.

OKAY – now about that bibliography....

AS SHOULD COME as no surprise, I kept receipts, so here are my citations.

These are the articles that informed my thinking last year. They're presented below in mostly chronological order, with the occasional comment. At the end I've collated a few links to additional articles that I didn't get to reference in this book, but which I still found useful and thought you might like.

I apologize that some of these are behind paywalls.

SHAH, Megha, et al. "Prevalence of and Factors Associated With Nurse Burnout in the US." JAMA Network, 4 Feb. 2021. https://jamanetwork.com/journals/jamanetworkopen/fullarticle/2775923

OFRI, Danielle. "Opinion | The Business of Health Care Depends on Exploiting Doctors and Nurses." The New York Times, 8 June 2019. NYTimes.com, https://www.nytimes.com/2019/06/08/opinion/sunday/hospitals-doctors-nurses-burnout.html.

. . .

ITALIAN NEWS VIDEO from inside an ICU: Coronavirus, dentro il reparto di terapia intensiva. www.la7.it, 5 Mar. 2020. https://www.la7.it/piazzapulita/video/coronavirus-dentro-il-reparto-di-terapia-intensiva-05-03-2020-311522 . Accessed 13 June 2021.

GREEN, Jason & Kelliher, Fiona. "Three San Jose TSA Agents Test Positive COVID-19, but Exposure to Travelers Remains Unknown." The Mercury News, 11 Mar. 2020, https://www.mercurynews.com/2020/03/10/san-jose-three-tsa-agents-test-positive-for-covid-19.

LANDSVERK, Gabby. "The CDC Says Healthcare Workers Who Can't Get a Mask Should Use a Bandana or Scarf as a 'last Resort' as Supplies Run Short." Business Insider, 19 Mar. 2020.https://www.businessinsider.com/cdc-recommends-health-workers-use-bandanas-face-masks-crisis-2020-3. Accessed 13 June 2021.

WASHINGTON POST. "Perspective | Doctors and Nurses Are Already Feeling the Psychic Shock of Treating the Coronavirus." www.washingtonpost.com, 18 Mar. 2020. https://www.washingtonpost.com/outlook/2020/03/18/doctors-nurses-are-already-feeling-psychic-shock-treating-coronavirus/. Accessed 14 June 2021.

BRUER, Wes & Matthew Hilk. "Despite Federal Guidelines, Trump Suggests 'sanitizing' and Reusing Medical Masks." CNN, 21 Mar. 2020. https://www.cnn.com/2020/03/21/politics/trump-sanitize-medical-masks/index.html. Accessed 13 June 2021.

· · ·

KNODEL, Jamie. "Texas Lt. Gov.: Grandparents Aren't Afraid to Die for Economy." NBC News, 24 Mar. 2020. https://www.nbcnews.com/news/us-news/texas-lt-gov-dan-patrick-suggests-he-other-seniors-willing-n1167341. Accessed 13 June 2021.

WISE, Justin. "Kudlow Says US Will Have to Make 'difficult Trade-offs' on Coronavirus: 'Cure Can't Be Worse than Disease.'" The Hill, 23 Mar. 2020, https://thehill.com/homenews/administration/489064-kudlow-says-us-will-have-to-make-difficult-trade-offs-on-coronavirus.

BREUNINGER, KEVIN. "TRUMP WANTS 'PACKED CHURCHES' and Economy Open Again on Easter Despite the Deadly Threat of Coronavirus." CNBC, 24 Mar. 2020, https://www.cnbc.com/2020/03/24/coronavirus-response-trump-wants-to-reopen-us-economy-by-easter.html.

DALE, Daniel (@ddale8)."https://Twitter.Com/Ddale8/Status/1245843578443706369." Twitter, https://twitter.com/ddale8/status/1245843578443706369. Accessed 13 June 2021. [CA: this was in regard to Trump's, 'We're not an ordering clerk' comment. @ddale8 faithfully transcribed all of Trump's pressers for the entire presidency, I believe.]

LEVEY, Noam. "Hospitals Say Feds Are Seizing Masks and Other Coronavirus Supplies without a Word." Los Angeles Times, 7 Apr. 2020, https://www.latimes.com/politics/story/2020-04-07/hospitals-washington-seize-coronavirus-supplies.

. . .

KISSLER, Stephen M., et al. "Projecting the Transmission Dynamics of SARS-CoV-2 through the Postpandemic Period." Science, vol. 368, no. 6493, May 2020, pp. 860–68. science.sciencemag.org, doi:10.1126/science.abb5793.

BEAUCHAMP, Zack. "A Disturbing New Study Suggests Sean Hannity's Show Helped Spread the Coronavirus." Vox, 22 Apr. 2020, https://www.vox.com/policy-and-politics/2020/4/22/21229360/coronavirus-covid-19-fox-news-sean-hannity-misinformation-death.

BBC. "Coronavirus: Outcry after Trump Suggests Injecting Disinfectant as Treatment." BBC News, 24 Apr. 2020. www.bbc.com, https://www.bbc.com/news/world-us-canada-52407177.

KAPLAN, Sheila. "F.D.A. Orders Companies to Submit Antibody Test Data." The New York Times, 4 May 2020. NYTimes.com, https://www.nytimes.com/2020/05/04/health/fda-antibody-tests-coronavirus.html.

OPRYSKO, Caitlyn. "Trump Drafts Everyday Americans to Adopt His Battlefield Rhetoric." POLITICO, 9 May 2020. https://www.politico.com/news/2020/05/09/donald-trump-coronavirus-wartime-rhetoric-245566. Accessed 13 June 2021.

KAITLAN COLLINS AND PETER MORRIS. "One of Trump's Personal Valets Has Tested Positive for Coronavirus." CNN, 7 May 2020. https://www.cnn.com/2020/05/07/politics/trump-valet-tests-positive-covid-19/index.html. Accessed 13 June 2021.

. . .

KAISER HEALTH NEWS. "All West Wing Employees Will Be Required to Wear Masks After Outbreak Scare At White House." 12 May 2020, https://khn.org/morning-breakout/all-west-wing-employees-will-be-required-to-wear-masks-after-outbreak-scare-at-white-house/.

PEREZ, Matt. "Trump on Healthcare Workers: 'They're Running into Death Just Like Soldiers Run Into Bullets.'" Forbes, 14 May 2020. https://www.forbes.com/sites/mattperez/2020/05/14/trump-on-healthcare-workers-theyre-running-into-death-just-like-soldiers-run-into-bullets/. Accessed 13 June 2021.

MELLO, Michelle, et al. "Attacks on Public Health Officials During Covid-19." JAMA Network, 5 Aug. 2020. https://jamanetwork.com/journals/jama/fullarticle/2769291

FURUSE, Yuki, et al. "Clusters of Coronavirus Disease in Communities, Japan, January–April 2020." Volume 26, Number 9—September 2020 - Emerging Infectious Diseases Journal - CDC. wwwnc.cdc.gov, doi:10.3201/eid2609.202272. Accessed 13 June 2021.

WU, Katherine J. "2 Stylists Had Coronavirus, but Wore Masks. 139 Clients Didn't Fall Sick." The New York Times, 14 July 2020. NYTimes.com, https://www.nytimes.com/2020/07/14/health/coronavirus-hair-salon-masks.html.

. . .

HOEVEN, Emily. "Newsom: All Californians Must Wear Masks." CalMatters, 19 June 2020, https://calmatters.org/newsletters/whatmatters/2020/06/gavin-newsom-face-masks-california/.

HENG, Larry. "'We Will Send Police. With Flame-Throwers': Italian Mayors Lose It at People Refusing to Self Isolate." National Post, 23 Mar. 2020. https://nationalpost.com/news/world/we-will-send-police-with-flame-throwers-italian-mayors-lose-it-at-people-refusing-to-self-isolate. Accessed 13 June 2021.

HEALTHLINE. "Black Lives Matter Protests Didn't Contribute to the COVID-19 Surge." 8 July 2020, https://www.healthline.com/health-news/black-lives-matter-protests-didnt-contribute-to-covid19-surge.

HANSEN, Sarah. "A National Mask Mandate Could Save The U.S. Economy $1 Trillion, Goldman Sachs Says." Forbes, 30 June 2020. https://www.forbes.com/sites/sarahhansen/2020/06/30/a-national-mask-mandate-could-save-the-us-economy-1-trillion-goldman-sachs-says/. Accessed 14 June 2021.

    Neal, David. "Florida Reports 15, 300 New Cases—A Record for One Day Anywhere in the U.S." Miami Herald, 20 July 2020. https://www.miamiherald.com/news/coronavirus/article244173462.html. (CA: re: Disney World reopening right as Florida reports a one-day record for the entire US)

BEGLEY, Sharon. "Trump Said Covid-19 Testing 'creates More Cases.' We Did the Math." STAT, 20 July 2020. https://www.

statnews.com/2020/07/20/trump-said-more-covid19-testing-creates-more-cases-we-did-the-math/.

REINBERG, Steven. "Sweden's COVID Policy Didn't Create Herd Immunity." WebMD, 13 Aug. 2020. https://www.webmd.com/lung/news/20200813/swedens-no-lockdown-policy-didnt-achieve-herd-immunity. Accessed 13 June 2021.

FIORE, Kristina. "The Cost of Herd Immunity in the U.S." Medpage Today, 1 Sept. 2020, https://www.medpagetoday.com/infectiousdisease/covid19/88401.

ECARMA, Caleb. "DHS Says It's 'Working on' a Black Lives Matter Crackdown." Vanity Fair, 1 Sept. 2020. https://www.vanityfair.com/news/2020/09/dhs-chad-wolf-working-on-black-lives-matter-crackdown. Accessed 13 June 2021.

HOLMAN, Curt. "Former GOP Candidate Herman Cain Dies of COVID-19." WebMD, 30 July 2020. https://www.webmd.com/lung/news/20200730/herman-cain-dies-of-covid19. Accessed 13 June 2021.

DIAMOND, Jeremy, Kristen Holmes, and Dr. Sanjay Gupta. "Fauci Says He Was in Surgery When Task Force Discussed CDC Testing Guidelines." CNN, 27 Aug. 2020. https://www.cnn.com/2020/08/26/politics/fauci-coronavirus-cdc-testing/index.html. Accessed 13 June 2021.

. . .

GUMBRECHT, Jamie, Jen Christensen, Elizabeth Cohen and Naomi Thomas. "CDC Abruptly Removes Guidance about Airborne Coronavirus Transmission, Says Update 'Was Posted in Error.'" CNN, 20 Sept. 2020. https://www.cnn.com/2020/09/21/health/cdc-reverts-airborne-transmission-guidance/index.html. Accessed 13 June 2021.

GESSEN, Masha. "The President Is Shilling Beans." The New Yorker, 16 July, 2020. https://www.newyorker.com/news/our-columnists/the-president-is-shilling-beans. Accessed 13 June 2021.

O'KANE, Caitlin. "Trump Said Coronavirus 'Affects Virtually Nobody,' as U.S. Surpasses 200,000 Deaths." CBS News, 22 Sept. 2021. https://www.cbsnews.com/news/covid-it-affects-virutally-nobody-trump-coronavirus-rally/. Accessed 13 June 2021.

BRANSWELL, Helen. "President Trump Has Tested Positive for Coronavirus." STAT, 2 Oct. 2020, https://www.statnews.com/2020/10/02/trump-coronavirus-positive-melania/.

WALKER, Molly. "HCQ No Longer Approved Even a Little for COVID-19." Medpage Today, 15 June 2020, https://www.medpagetoday.com/infectiousdisease/covid19/87066.

NEUMAN, Scott. "Man Dies, Woman Hospitalized After Taking Form Of Chloroquine To Prevent COVID-19." NPR.Org, 24 Mar. 2020. https://www.npr.org/sections/coronavirus-live-updates/2020/03/24/820512107/man-dies-woman-hospitalized-after-taking-form-of-chloroquine-to-prevent-covid-19. Accessed 13 June 2021.

. . .

SPENCER, Craig (@Craig_A_Spencer). "https://Twitter.-Com/Craig_a_spencer/Status/1312782277005455362." Twitter, 4 Oct. 2020. https://twitter.com/craig_a_spencer/status/1312782277005455362. Accessed 13 June 2021. [CA: re: Trump not wearing a mask while infectious with covid.]

SHEPHERD, KATIE. "'EPIDEMIOLOGISTS JUST WANNA VOMIT': Doctors Disturbed after Trump Removes His Mask at the White House." Washington Post, 6 Oct. 2020. www.washingtonpost.com, https://www.washingtonpost.com/nation/2020/10/06/trump-coronavirus-mask-doctors/. Accessed 13 June 2021.

RUPAR, Aaron (@atrupar). Twitter, 6 Oct. 2020. https://twitter.com/atrupar/status/1313553163354624006. Accessed 13 June 2021. [CA: fuckin' Fox.]

SWAN, Jonathan. "Trump Launches Multimillion-Dollar Ad Campaign Aimed at Winning Back Seniors." Axios, 12 Oct. 2020. https://www.axios.com/trump-multimillion-ad-campaign-senior-citizens-e185216f-3b72-4995-afb1-46f2d30fea9c.html. Accessed 13 June 2021.

"COVID-19 VACCINE from Pfizer and BioNTech Is Strongly Effective, Data Show." STAT, 9 Nov. 2020, https://www.statnews.com/2020/11/09/covid-19-vaccine-from-pfizer-and-biontech-is-strongly-effective-early-data-from-large-trial-indicate/.

. . .

REIMANN, Nicholas. "Tulsa Has Run Out Of ICU Beds And El Paso Is Out Of Morgue Space—Here's The Latest Grim Toll Of Covid." Forbes, 10 Nov. 2020. https://www.forbes.com/sites/ nicholasreimann/2020/11/10/tulsa-has-run-out-of-icu-beds-and-el- paso-is-out-of-morgue-space-heres-the-latest-grim-toll-of-covid/. Accessed 13 June 2021.

RENWICK, Danielle. "Anger After North Dakota Governor Asks COVID-Positive Health Staff to Stay on Job." Kaiser Health News, 18 Nov. 2020, https://khn.org/news/anger-after-north-dakota- governor-asks-covid-positive-health-staff-to-stay-on-job/.

ASMELASH, Leah and Konstantin Toropin. "Utah Sent Every Phone in the State an Emergency Alert Warning about Rapidly Rising Covid-19 Cases and Overwhelmed Hospitals." CNN, 30 Oct. 2020. https://www.cnn.com/2020/10/30/us/utah-emergency-alert- covid-19-trnd/index.html. Accessed 13 June 2021.

NURSEKELSEY (@NURSEKELSEY). "https://Twitter.- Com/Nursekelsey/Status/1325889278166110210." Twitter, 9 Nov. 2020. https://twitter.com/nursekelsey/status/ 1325889278166110210. Accessed 13 June 2021. [CA: regarding the extra staff demand covid puts on hospitals.]

KAISER HEALTH NEWS. "Sturgis Biker Rally Linked To 260,000 COVID Cases." 9 Sept. 2020, https://khn.org/morning-breakout/ sturgis-biker-rally-linked-to-260000-covid-cases/.

. . .

KCTV KANSAS CITY. "KC Metro 'Now Reached Uncontrolled Community Spread of COVID.'" 10 Nov. 2020. https://www.kctv5.com/coronavirus/kc-metro-now-reached-uncontrolled-community-spread-of-covid/article_10c979ec-23b9-11eb-b8bo-fb946f4c40ff.html. Accessed 13 June 2021.

SMITH, Mitch, et al. "More than 1 in 400 Americans Test Positive in a Week, Pushing New Jersey to a Record and Prompting Restrictions in North Dakota." The New York Times, 13 Nov. 2020. NYTimes.com, https://www.nytimes.com/2020/11/14/world/more-than-1-in-400-americans-test-positive-in-a-week-pushing-new-jersey-to-a-record-and-prompting-restrictions-in-north-dakota.html.

MAYER, Eric. "KOTG: South Dakota Surpasses 2,000 New Coronavirus Cases in a Day, Canton Hit Hard by COVID-19 and Spearfish Promotes Mask Wearing." KELOLAND.Com, 13 Nov. 2020, https://www.keloland.com/on-the-go/kotg-south-dakota-surpasses-2000-new-coronavirus-cases-in-a-day-canton-hit-hard-by-covid-19-and-spearfish-promotes-mask-wearing/.

YONG, Ed. "'No One Is Listening to Us.'" The Atlantic, 13 Nov. 2020, https://www.theatlantic.com/health/archive/2020/11/third-surge-breaking-healthcare-workers/617091/. [CA: re: Iowa's ICU bed situation.]

MOLTENI, Megan. "Iowa's Covid Wave and the Limits of Personal Responsibility." Wired, 20 Nov. 2020. www.wired.com, https://www.wired.com/story/iowas-covid-wave-and-the-limits-of-personal-responsibility. Accessed 13 June 2021.

· · ·

LAS CRUCES SUN-NEWS. "New Mexico Shelter-in-Place Order Issued to Mitigate Coronavirus Spread." 13 Nov. 2020. https://www.lcsun-news.com/story/news/2020/11/13/new-mexico-shelter-in-place-order-covid-cases-increase/6283724002/. Accessed 13 June 2021.

ZENGERLE, Patricia and Steve Holland,. "Trump's Vaccine Team Will Not Brief Biden Administration: U.S Senators." Reuters, 19 Nov. 2020. www.reuters.com, https://www.reuters.com/article/us-usa-election-vaccine-idUSKBN27Z2UA.

CBS NEWS. "Nevada Governor Issues Three-Week 'Statewide Pause' as Coronavirus Cases Rise." 23 Nov. 2020. https://www.cbsnews.com/news/nevada-covid-statewide-pause-governor-sisolak/. Accessed 13 June 2021.

CLEAVON MD (@CLEAVON_MD). "https://Twitter.-Com/Cleavon_md/Status/1330896313551085574." Twitter, 23 Nov. 2020. https://twitter.com/cleavon_md/status/1330896313551085574. Accessed 14 June 2021. [CA: This is a doctor, venting his frustration that whatever ICU beds the government claims there are in Arizona appear to be imaginary.]

TAVERNISE, Sabrina. "Grim Day in U.S. as Covid-19 Deaths and Hospitalizations Set Records." The New York Times, 3 Dec. 2020. NYTimes.com, https://www.nytimes.com/live/2020/12/02/world/covid-19-coronavirus.

. . .

BUDRYK, Zack. "US Reports 3,100 COVID-19 Deaths in One Day, Surpassing Previous Record by 20 Percent." The Hill, 3 Dec. 2020, https://thehill.com/policy/healthcare/528519-us-marks-record-number-of-covid-19-deaths-in-one-day.

LAFRANIERE, Sharon, et al. "Trump Administration Officials Passed When Pfizer Offered Months Ago to Sell the U.S. More Vaccine Doses." The New York Times, 7 Dec. 2020. NYTimes.com, https://www.nytimes.com/2020/12/07/us/trump-covid-vaccine-pfizer.html.

ELLIS, Ralph. "British Woman First to Get Pfizer COVID-19 Vaccine." WebMD, 8 Dec. 2020. https://www.webmd.com/vaccines/covid-19-vaccine/news/20201208/british-woman-first-to-get-pfizer-covid-19-vaccine. Accessed 14 June 2021.

JORDAN, Jim (@Jim_Jordan). Twitter, 8 Dec. 2020. https://twitter.com/jim_jordan/status/1336420640291688457. Accessed 14 June 2021. [CA: Jim Jordan, ladies and gentlemen, in his own words.]

CDC. "CASES, DATA, AND SURVEILLANCE." Centers for Disease Control and Prevention, 11 Feb. 2020, https://www.cdc.gov/coronavirus/2019-ncov/covid-data/investigations-discovery/hospitalization-death-by-race-ethnicity.html.

DANA, Joe. "Yuma Doctor Receives Personal Thanks from Joe Biden for COVID-19 Work." 12news.com, 7 Dec. 2020. https://www.12news.com/article/news/local/valley/yuma-doctor-receives-personal-thanks-from-joe-biden-for-covid-19-work/75-c6268f62-efc9-4598-9c6b-8f934896623f. Accessed 14 June 2021.

LEATHERBY, Lauren, et al. "'There's No Place for Them to Go': I.C.U. Beds Near Capacity Across U.S." The New York Times, 9 Dec. 2020. NYTimes.com, https://www.nytimes.com/interactive/2020/12/09/us/covid-hospitals-icu-capacity.html.

MANJOO, Farhad. "Opinion: I Traced My Covid-19 Bubble and It's Enormous." The New York Times, 20 Nov. 2020. NYTimes.com, https://www.nytimes.com/2020/11/20/opinion/sunday/covid-bubble-thanksgiving-family.html.

MANJOO, Farhad. "Opinion: The Hidden 'Fourth Wave' of the Pandemic." The New York Times, 9 Dec. 2020. NYTimes.com, https://www.nytimes.com/2020/12/09/opinion/coronavirus-mental-health.html.

MADANI, Doha. "First Trucks with Covid-19 Vaccine Roll out of Pfizer Plant in Michigan." NBC News, 13 Dec. 2020. https://www.nbcnews.com/news/us-news/first-trucks-covid-19-vaccine-roll-out-pfizer-plant-michigan-n1251037. Accessed 14 June 2021.

MULCAHY, SHAWN, ET AL. "TEXAS' ICU Capacity Is the Lowest since the Start of the Pandemic." ABC13 Houston, 14 Dec. 2020, https://abc13.com/8771103/.

. . .

GITTLESON, Ben. "White House Security Director Has Part of Leg Amputated after Falling Severely Ill with COVID-19, Fundraiser Says." ABC News, 16 Dec. 2020. https://abcnews.go.com/Politics/white-house-security-director-part-leg-amputated-falling/story?id=74757679. Accessed 14 June 2021.

THE GUARDIAN. "Two People Dying Every Hour in Los Angeles County as It Sees 'Explosive Surge.'" 17 Dec. 2020, http://www.theguardian.com/us-news/2020/dec/17/covid-los-angeles-county-two-people-dying-every-hour.

KILGORE, Tomi. "U.S. COVID-19 Death Toll Jumps to Daily Record of More than 3,600, and Hospitalizations Extend Record Streak." MarketWatch, 17 Dec. 2020. https://www.marketwatch.com/story/u-s-covid-19-death-toll-jumps-to-daily-record-of-more-than-3-600-and-hospitalizations-extend-record-streak-11608221484. Accessed 14 June 2021.

PAPENFUSS, Mary. "Millions Of COVID-19 Vaccine Doses Stuck in Warehouses Until Federal Orders, Pfizer Says." HuffPost, 17 Dec. 2020,   https://www.huffpost.com/entry/pfizer-warehouse-doses-trump-administration_n_5fdbe0c4c5b6094c0ff08c4a.

MARTINEZ, Lita. "Southern California Has Run Out Of ICU Beds For Coronavirus Patients." LAist, 18 Dec. 2020, https://laist.com/news/icu-capacity-runs-out-socal-coronavirus-patients.

LI, Kenneth. "Murdoch Receives COVID-19 Vaccine as Fox News Host Casts Suspicion on Campaign." Reuters, 18 Dec.

2020. www.reuters.com, https://www.reuters.com/article/us-health-coronavirus-murdoch-idUSKBN28S2J7.

GUO, Eileen and Karen Hao. "This Is the Stanford Vaccine Algorithm That Left out Frontline Doctors." MIT Technology Review, 21 Dec. 2020. https://www.technologyreview.com/2020/12/21/1015303/stanford-vaccine-algorithm/. Accessed 14 June 2021.

ABC7.COM. "Video of Kirk Cameron Maskless Caroling Event in Thousand Oaks." ABC7 Los Angeles, 23 Dec. 2020, https://abc7.com/8996273/.

CAMBERG, Nicki, et al. "Analysis & Updates: In the Deadliest Month Yet, the Pandemic Is Regional Again: This Week in COVID-19 Data, Dec 23." The COVID Tracking Project, 23 Dec. 2020. https://covidtracking.com/analysis-updates/deadliest-month-yet-pandemic-regional-again-dec-23. Accessed 14 June 2021.

KESLING, Ben. "Wisconsin Pharmacist Sentenced to Three Years in Prison for Tampering With Covid Vaccines." Wall Street Journal, 8 June 2021. www.wsj.com, https://www.wsj.com/articles/wisconsin-pharmacist-sentenced-to-three-years-in-prison-for-tampering-with-covid-vaccines-11623186447.

MIDDLE EAST MONITOR. "Egypt: Entire ICU Ward Dies after Oxygen Supply Fails." 4 Jan. 2021, https://www.middleeastmonitor.com/20210104-egypt-entire-icu-ward-dies-after-oxygen-supply-fails/.

. . .

NIRAPPIL, Fenit and William Wan. "Los Angeles Is Running out of Oxygen for Patients as Covid Hospitalizations Hit Record Highs Nationwide." Washington Post, 5 Jan. 2021. www.washingtonpost.com, https://www.washingtonpost.com/health/2021/01/05/covid-hospitalizations-los-angeles-oxygen/. Accessed 14 June 2021.

HOLMES, Kristen and Sara Murray. "Despite Trump Administration Promise, Government Has No More 'reserve' 2nd Vaccine Doses." CNN, 15 Jan. 2021. https://www.cnn.com/2021/01/15/politics/coronavirus-vaccine-reserve-dose/index.html. Accessed 14 June 2021.

HALTIWANGER, John. "More Americans Have Now Died from COVID-19 than the Number of US Troops Killed during World War II." Business Insider, 20 Jan. 2020. https://www.businessinsider.com/more-americans-dead-covid-19-us-battle-deaths-wwii-2020-12. Accessed 14 June 2021.

THE COVID TRACKING PROJECT. "National Data: Deaths." https://covidtracking.com/data/national/deaths. Accessed 14 June 2021.

GERBER, Marissa and Irfan Khan. "Dodger Stadium's COVID-19 Vaccination Site Temporarily Shut down after Protesters Gather at Entrance." Los Angeles Times, 30 Jan. 2021, https://www.latimes.com/california/story/2021-01-30/dodger-stadiums-covid-19-vaccination-site-shutdown-after-dozens-of-protesters-gather-at-entrance.

. . .

ACOSTA, Jim and Caroline Kelly. "Donald and Melania Trump Received Covid Vaccine at the White House in January." CNN, 1 Mar. 2021. https://www.cnn.com/2021/03/01/politics/trump-melania-vaccinated-white-house/index.html. Accessed 14 June 2021.

GRISALES, Claudia. "Rep. Ron Wright Is 1st Member of Congress To Die After Coronavirus Diagnosis." NPR.org, 8 Feb. 2021. https://www.npr.org/2021/02/08/965370870/1st-member-of-congress-texas-rep-ron-wright-dies-following-covid-19-diagnosis. Accessed 14 June 2021.

VAZQUEZ, Maegan. "Biden Declares There Will Be Enough Vaccines for 300 Million Americans by End of July." CNN, 11 Feb. 2021. https://www.cnn.com/2021/02/11/politics/joe-biden-vaccine-distribution-trump-administration/index.html. Accessed 14 June 2021.

OFFICE OF THE TEXAS GOVERNOR. "Governor Abbott Lifts Mask Mandate, Opens Texas 100 Percent." 2 Mar. 2021. https://gov.texas.gov/news/post/governor-abbott-lifts-mask-mandate-opens-texas-100-percent. Accessed 14 June 2021.

BBC NEWS, "Kate Garraway: 'My Husband Is Devastated by Covid.'" 23 May, 2021. www.bbc.com, https://www.bbc.com/news/av/uk-57218737. Accessed 14 June 2021.

ORTIZ, Jorge L. "'Blood on His Hands': As US Surpasses 400,000 COVID-19 Deaths, Experts Blame Trump Administration for a 'pre-

ventable' Loss of Life." USA TODAY, 17 Jan. 2021. https://www.
usatoday.com/story/news/nation/2021/01/17/covid-19-us-400-
000-deaths-experts-blame-trump-administration/6642685002/.
Accessed 14 June 2021.

WAN, William. "Burned out by the Pandemic, 3 in 10 Health-Care
Workers Consider Leaving the Profession." Washington Post, 22
Apr. 2021, https://www.washingtonpost.com/health/2021/04/22/
health-workers-covid-quit/.

NAST, Condé. "Tucker Carlson, Who Shouldn't Be Allowed Within
2,000 Feet of Playgrounds, Tells Viewers to Call Child Protective
Services on People Whose Kids Wear Masks." Vanity Fair, https://
www.vanityfair.com/news/2021/04/tucker-carlson-masks-child-
protective-services. Accessed 6 July 2021.

HELSEL, Phil and Austin Mullen. "Covid Has Claimed More than
600,000 Lives in United States." NBC News, 3 Jun. 2021. https://
www.nbcnews.com/news/us-news/covid-has-claimed-more-600-
000-lives-united-states-n1269580. Accessed 14 June 2021.

NEWS WIRES. "France to Honour Health Workers Killed by
Covid-19 with Special Status." France 24, 21 May 2021, https://
www.france24.com/en/france/20210521-france-to-honour-health-
workers-killed-by-covid-19-with-special-status.

SPENCER, Jane, The Guardian, and Christina Jewett. "12 Months
of Trauma: More Than 3,600 US Health Workers Died in Covid's

First Year." Kaiser Health News, 8 Apr. 2021, https://khn.org/news/article/us-health-workers-deaths-covid-lost-on-the-frontline/.

SILVERMAN, Rosa. "Vaccinated but Won't Go out? The Rise of Covid Anxiety Syndrome." The Telegraph, 3 May 2021. www.telegraph.co.uk,   https://www.telegraph.co.uk/health-fitness/mind/vaccinated-wont-go-rise-covid-anxiety-syndrome/.

INSTITUTE FOR HEALTH Metrics and Evaluation. "Estimation of Total Mortality Due to COVID-19." 22 Apr. 2021, http://www.healthdata.org/special-analysis/estimation-excess-mortality-due-covid-19-and-scalars-reported-covid-19-deaths.

MOZES, Alan. "Nurses Are Dying From Suicide at Higher Rates." WebMD, 14 Apr. 2021. https://www.webmd.com/lung/news/20210414/nurses-are-dying-from-suicide-at-higher-rates. Accessed 14 June 2021.

VAUGHN, Natalie. "Nurse Turnover Rates: How to Reduce Health-care Turnover." Relias, 27 Oct. 2020, https://www.rclias.com/blog/how-to-reduce-healthcare-turnover.

TUNG, Liz. "Why Mandated Nurse-to-Patient Ratios Have Become One of the Most Controversial Ideas in Health Care." WHYY, 29 Nov. 2019. https://whyy.org/segments/why-mandated-nurse-to-patient-ratios-have-become-one-of-the-most-controversial-ideas-in-health-care/. Accessed 14 June 2021.

. . .

ANDRZEJEWSKI, Adam. "Top U.S. 'Non-Profit' Hospitals & CEOs Are Racking Up Huge Profits." Forbes, 26 Jun. 2019. https://www.forbes.com/sites/adamandrzejewski/2019/06/26/top-u-s-non-profit-hospitals-ceos-are-racking-up-huge-profits/. Accessed 14 June 2021.

GANGEL, Jamie, Brian Stelter, and Michael Warren. "Pence Signs a Seven-Figure Book Deal, but Trump and Other Administration Alums Face a Tough Market in Publishing." CNN, 7 Apr. 2021. https://www.cnn.com/2021/04/07/politics/pence-book-deal-trump-administration/index.html. Accessed 14 June 2021.

MCCALL, Rosie. "From 'Smoking Doesn't Kill' to Conversion Therapy—Mike Pence's Most Controversial Science Remarks." Newsweek, 27 Feb. 2020, https://www.newsweek.com/mike-pence-coronavirus-science-hiv-aids-smoking-evolution-climate-change-1489458.

ADDITIONAL ARTICLES W/SOME more commentary:

STAFF, Media Matters. "Sean Hannity Reads Mike Pence a Letter from Unidentified Doctor Detailing a Drug 'Regimen' the Doctor Claims Prevents Coronavirus Deaths." Media Matters for America, 23 Mar. 2020. https://www.mediamatters.org/sean-hannity/sean-hannity-reads-mike-pence-letter-unidentified-doctor-detailing-drug-regimen-doctor. Accessed 14 June 2021.

· · ·

EXPLAIN to me again why the fuck this happened? Like either of them knew anything about fucking medicine in the least, and how this wasn't dangerous and actionable? The second this fucking nonsense went on the air, someone somewhere should've turned the lights off in their studio.

Fucking murderers.

Meanwhile, in fact-land: The Atlantic had stellar journalism the entire time, and Ed Yong heartily deserves the Pulitzer he just won. I am writing my story about my experiences with covid, but he will be the one to write *the story* about it, I feel.

YONG, Ed. "America Is About to Choose How Bad the Pandemic Will Get." The Atlantic, 28 Oct. 2020, https://www.theatlantic.com/health/archive/2020/10/coronavirus-election/616884/.

YONG, Ed. "Hospitals Know What's Coming." The Atlantic, 20 Nov. 2020, https://www.theatlantic.com/health/archive/2020/11/americas-best-prepared-hospital-nearly-overwhelmed/617156/.

YONG, Ed. "'No One Is Listening to Us.'" The Atlantic, 13 Nov. 2020, https://www.theatlantic.com/health/archive/2020/11/third-surge-breaking-healthcare-workers/617091/.

THIS WAS my favorite graph to send to people to explain spread in the beginning—it's just a really great graphic for what went on:

REUTERS. "2019 CORONAVIRUS: THE KOREAN CLUSTERS." 20 Mar. 2020, https://graphics.reuters.com/CHINA-

HEALTH-SOUTHKOREA-CLUSTERS/0100B5G33SB/
index.html. Accessed 14 June 2021.

BANKERS LOOKING to cash out on suppling PPE (are you surprised? And, again, BILLIONAIRE PHILANTHROPY IS A MYTH. They provide nothing that adequate taxation couldn't!)

FANG, Lee. "Banks Pressure Health Care Firms to Raise Prices on Critical Drugs, Medical Supplies for Coronavirus." The Intercept, 19 Mar. 2020. https://theintercept.com/2020/03/19/coronavirus-vaccine-medical-supplies-price-gouging/. Accessed 14 June 2021.

EARLY MATH ON ICU BED/VENTILATOR capacity, from March 2020:

HALPERN, Neil A. and Kay See Tan. "United States Resource Availability for COVID-19." Society of Critical Care Medicine (SCCM), 13 Mar. 2020. https://sccm.org/Blog/March-2020/United-States-Resource-Availability-for-COVID-19. Accessed 14 June 2021.

BORIS JOHNSON'S former aide rats him out for covid deaths.
   BBC News. "Dominic Cummings: Thousands Died Needlessly after Covid Mistakes." 26 May 2021. www.bbc.com, https://www.bbc.com/news/uk-politics-57253578.

⎯ᴗ⎯ᴗ⎯

MORE ARTICLES ABOUT COGNITIVE DISSONANCE, PTSD, and the danger healthcare workers are in (and have been in, this whole damn time.)

RANNEY, Megan and Jessi Gold. "Doctors: Health Care Workers Are Experiencing More than Covid-19 Burnout." CNN, 18 Nov. 2020. https://www.cnn.com/2020/11/18/opinions/health-care-workers-covid-19-burnout-ranney-gold/index.html. Accessed 14 June 2021.

HOFFMAN, Jan. "'I Can't Turn My Brain Off': PTSD and Burnout Threaten Medical Workers." The New York Times, 16 May 2020. NYTimes.com, https://www.nytimes.com/2020/05/16/health/coronavirus-ptsd-medical-workers.html.

JOHNSON, Sarah et al. "'They Stormed the ICU and Beat the Doctor': Health Workers under Attack." The Guardian, 7 June 2021, http://www.theguardian.com/global-development/2021/jun/07/they-stormed-the-icu-and-beat-the-doctor-health-workers-under-attack.

JOHNSON, Sarah. "Spat at, Abused, Attacked: Healthcare Staff Face Rising Violence during Covid." The Guardian, 7 June 2021, http://www.theguardian.com/global-development/2021/jun/07/spat-at-abused-attacked-healthcare-staff-face-rising-violence-during-covid.

. . .

AND HERE'S why they're doing it: because they don't share the same reality as we do, and so when our reality wins BECAUSE COVID IS REAL, AND THEIR ACTIONS ARE KILLING PEOPLE, they get violent.

And yet we still fucking try to save them....

VINOPAL, Lauren. "The Nurses Working to Save Coronavirus Deniers." MEL Magazine, 17 Aug. 2020, https://melmagazine.com/en-us/story/the-nurses-working-to-save-coronavirus-deniers.

I MEAN, these people are fucking invested in their delusions:

VILLEGAS, Paulina. "South Dakota Nurse Says Many Patients Deny the Coronavirus Exists—Right up until Death." Washington Post, 16 Nov. 2020. www.washingtonpost.com, https://www.washingtonpost.com/health/2020/11/16/south-dakota-nurse-coronavirus-deniers/. Accessed 14 June 2021.

MEANWHILE, ED RNs are experiencing PTSD at twice the rate of doctors:

TRUDGILL, Diane I. N., et al. "Prevalent Posttraumatic Stress Disorder among Emergency Department Personnel: Rapid Systematic Review." Humanities and Social Sciences Communications, vol. 7, no. 1, Sept. 2020, pp. 1–7. https://www.nature.com/articles/s41599-020-00584-x, doi:10.1057/s41599-020-00584-x.

SOME SAD STATS on both ends of the age range:

NANIA, Rachel. "95 Percent of Americans Killed by COVID Were 50+." AARP, 1 Apr. 2021. https://www.aarp.org/health/conditions-treatments/info-2020/coronavirus-deaths-older-adults.html. Accessed 14 June 2021.

JENCO, Melissa. "Children Make up Nearly 21% of New COVID-19 Cases." AAP News, 19 Apr. 2021. www.aappublications.org, https://www.aappublications.org/news/2021/04/19/pediatric-covid-cases-041921.

ROUGHLY 300 KIDS have died from covid. (And if you say, 'that's not too many', you need to go to the bathroom and wash your mouth out with soap. Or look your kid in the eye and say, 'Wellllllllllll....')

FOR PEOPLE who doubt we were merely treated like a commodity:

CHOI, Dan (@drdanchoi). Twitter, 22 Mar. 2020. https://twitter.com/drdanchoi/status/1241958791329067009.
    Accessed 14 June 2021.

THIS HAPPENED IN MULTIPLE LOCATIONS. Last year, during the first wave, hospitals would rather have 'not scared' people than protect us.

. . .

MEANWHILE, we had to deal with shit like this:

CORBEN, Billy (@BillyCorben). "https://Twitter.Com/Billycorben/Status/1241740081343447040." Twitter, 22 Mar. 2020. https://twitter.com/billycorben/status/1241740081343447040. Accessed 14 June 2021.

THIS IS film of a Florida County Commissioner saying you can kill coronavirus by blowing a hairdryer up your nose, and he learned it on OANN.

SO THERE WE were at work, listening to this bullshit, all the while knowing that if we got covid, or our loved ones got covid, while we might survive, we might also be in for a horrible long crawl back to our former health (and indeed, might never attain it).

LEES, Nathalie. "Researchers Are Closing in on Long Covid." The Economist, 29 Apr. 2021. The Economist, https://www.economist.com/science-and-technology/2021/04/29/researchers-are-closing-in-on-long-covid.

AND ONCE AGAIN, I want to point out that the United States wasted a TRILLION DOLLARS by not having a mask mandate:

ROSENBAUM, Leah. "The Hidden Costs of Coronavirus Hospitalizations." Forbes, 30 Oct. 2020. https://www.forbes.com/sites/leahrosenbaum/2020/10/30/the-hidden-costs-of-coronavirus-hospitalizations/. Accessed 14 June 2021.

. . .

ALL BECAUSE ASSHATS like Jared Kushner couldn't see the virtue in public health policy.

EBAN, Katherine. "How Jared Kushner's Secret Testing Plan 'Went Poof into Thin Air.'" Vanity Fair, 30 July 2020. https://www. vanityfair.com/news/2020/07/how-jared-kushners-secret-testing-plan-went-poof-into-thin-air. Accessed 15 June 2021.

AND TRUMP'S White House Chief of Staff couldn't be bothered to try to even control things....

SMITH, Allan. "'We're Not Going to Control the Pandemic,' Trump's Chief of Staff Says in Heated Interview." NBC News, 25 Oct. 2020. https://www.nbcnews.com/politics/donald-trump/meadows-says-we-re-not-going-control-pandemic-heated-interview-n1244681. Accessed 15 June 2021.

ALL THIS, even though even as early as March 20, 2020, laypeople (and hospital-people!) could see the writing on the wall and what was needed for us all to survive:

WARNER, Jason S. "The Sober Math Everyone Must Understand about the Pandemic." Medium, 20 Mar. 2020, https://medium. com/@Jason_Scott_Warner/the-sober-math-everyone-must-understand-about-the-pandemic-2b0145881993.

. . .

AND THEY ALWAYS KNEW THAT herd immunity was never an option, due to the mass casualties it would bring:

ASCHWANDEN, Christie. "The False Promise of Herd Immunity for COVID-19." Nature, vol. 587, no. 7832, Oct. 2020, pp. 26–28. https://www.nature.com/articles/d41586-020-02948-4:10.1038/d41586-020-02948-4.

PLEASE TRUST that I could go on and on, but my wrists are killing me—I've been working on this so hard I have to ice them every night.

THANK you all again for making it this far. I hope you got something out of the ride.
    —Cassie

Made in United States
North Haven, CT
19 March 2022

17312461R00232